T0129425

# Amazing You

By
Joanne Hammons

BALBOA.
PRESS
A DIVISION OF HAY HOUSE

Balboa Press books may be ordered through booksellers or by contacting:

Balboa Press
A Division of Hay House
1663 Liberty Drive
Bloomington, IN 47403
www.balboapress.com
1 (877) 407-4847

Because of the dynamic nature of the Internet, any web addresses or links contained in this book may have changed since publication and may no longer be valid. The views expressed in this work are solely those of the author and do not necessarily reflect the views of the publisher, and the publisher hereby disclaims any responsibility for them.

Scriptures taken from the Holy Bible, New International Version®, NIV®. Copyright © 1973, 1978, 1984, 2011 by Biblica, Inc.™ Used by permission of Zondervan. All rights reserved worldwide. www.zondervan.com The "NIV" and "New International Version" are trademarks registered in the United States Patent and Trademark Office by Biblica, Inc.™

The author of this book does not dispense medical advice or prescribe the use of any technique as a form of treatment for physical, emotional, or medical problems without the advice of a physician, either directly or indirectly. The intent of the author is only to offer information of a general nature to help you in your quest for emotional and spiritual well-being. In the event you use any of the information in this book for yourself, which is your constitutional right, the author and the publisher assume no responsibility for your actions.

Any people depicted in stock imagery provided by Thinkstock are models, and such images are being used for illustrative purposes only. Certain stock imagery © Thinkstock.

Print information available on the last page.

ISBN: 978-1-5043-9725-4 (sc)
ISBN: 978-1-5043-9727-8 (hc)
ISBN: 978-1-5043-9726-1 (e)

Library of Congress Control Number: 2018901407

Balboa Press rev. date: 02/09/2018

*A*mazing You will open your eyes to a new way of understanding how the body works and what it is telling you so that you can heal the cause and become your true authentic self.

# Dedications

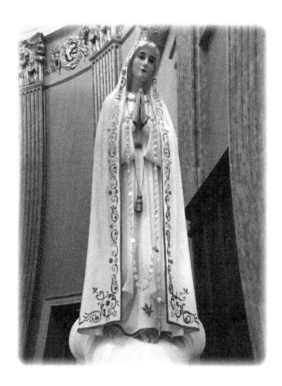

*I* dedicate this book to The Blessed Mother, who has always been
there for me and my family. To God, who loves us so much that He
sacrificed His Son Jesus to save us. To Jesus, who paid the ultimate
price for our sins so that we could go to heaven and to the Holy Spirit,
our counselor and our guide.

Also, I would like to thank my Healing Team, the Ascending Masters,
Archangels, Angels and the many Beings of Light that have protected
me, guided me, and helped me to heal. I am so very grateful for your
support and love. I thank you all.

# Contents

# Acknowledgments

I wish to acknowledge my parents who sacrificed so much for us 5 children to have the privilege of a Catholic Education. I am very grateful for all that you have done for me and my family and I love you two very much. To my loving husband and my two amazing sons, thank you for your support and unconditional love that you gave me through my healing journey, I love you and may God bless your lives always.

To Sr. Dorothy Merth who showed me how to become my true authentic self and taught me through love how to let go of fear and trust God. Sr. Dorothy was a true servant for our Lord. Through her healing practice she touched and changed so many lives including mine. Sr. Dorothy passed away at 100 years old on October 25, 2017. She never stopped serving God. She was truly a blessing to us all and will be missed greatly.

I am grateful for all the teachers in my life. They have come in many forms: my husband and children, parents, sisters, brothers, friends and acquaintances to name a few. I am grateful and thankful for all the lessons that we have share.

My gift to all of you is my book, "Amazing You". May you find the healing and help that you need to become your true authentic self.

With Love and Gratitude;
Joanne

> *"Oh, Lord my God, I cried to you for help, and you healed me." Psalm 30:2*

# Preface

This book will transform your life. Everything in this book are simple techniques and remedies that Sr. Dorothy and myself have used to help balance, remove and heal the energy blockages in our bodies. I will explain how the energy in your body works and how to clear the blockages in different ways. I will show you how to clear beliefs that are no longer serving you and how to move forward from them. I will explain and show you how to heal fears that are holding you back.

Through the Healing Mediation you will be able to clear energy blocks that are holding you back, blocks caused by traumas, abuse, childhood pain, unforgiveness, depression, anxiety, stress addictions and more.

I will also give you simple remedies to help your physical body to detox and heal.

Through your healing process your connection to God, Jesus, Holy Spirit, the Blessed Mother and your healing team and angels will become stronger and you will learn to hear that small voice inside of you that has always been there. Your body and I Am presence knows exactly what you need to heal. Your part is to listen to what your body is telling you and do it.

**"Be still and know that I am God". Psalm 46:10**

## About the Author

My name is Joan Hammons but everyone calls me Joanne. I have been working on people, teaching, writing, and co-creating healing techniques for over 20 years. The reason I started learning about alternative therapies is because I was sick with a Heart condition which caused numerous problems in my body at Age 17. I went for my college physical and they discovered a big problem with my heart. I was sent to the University of Minnesota for testing and was diagnosed as having Takayasu disease which is inflammation of the blood vessels leading out of the aorta. My disease was in the renal arteries. To make a long story short I had Angiogram with balloon dilatation and was put on a high dose of steroids to keep the inflammation down. I was going to school at the same time to be a Medical Lab Technician so I did my blood work and sent it to the doctors weekly. This went on for years and the steroids were taking a toll on my body. I was not able to keep anything down and my stomach hurt all the time. In my thirties I told my doctors that I couldn't do this anymore and I needed to find something that was going to heal me and not make me sick. My doctors said ok, and they would help me in whatever I want to do. The problem was that I didn't know what to do.

Back then I knew Jesus but never thought to ask Jesus for help, but he helped me through my dearest friend Beth. She introduced me to Sr. Dorothy and her alternative methods. When she told me about Sr. Dorothy I said to her, I am tired of doctors. She said, just go once. So I called Sr. Dorothy and got her answer machine. I left a message and said, I don't know why I am calling you because I don't even know what you can do for me. You can call me back if you want and left my number. After I hung up I said,

Ok God this is in your hands. If you want me to see Sr. Dorothy she is going to have to call me back. It wasn't even 10 seconds after I talked to God that Sr. Dorothy called me back and said, Joanne why don't you come in tomorrow and I said ok.

That day changed my life. I worked with Sr. Dorothy for 6 months and my stomach was healed. I was tapered off the steroids and blood pressure medicine and worked closely with my doctors and did my labs weekly. My disease has never come back. I am now 57 and have two beautiful, healthy sons after I was told that I couldn't have any children. Everything in this book has helped me to heal and I want to share it with you. My wish for you is that whatever is hurting you whether it is physical, emotional, spiritual or mental pain that you will find peace and healing. May God bless you and guide you on your journey.

# How can this book help you?

This book will give you the tools you need to help yourself, your families and friends. I will teach you many healing techniques and remedies that are simple and will have a profound effect on your physical body and the quality of your life. I know this because everything that I will share with you has helped me, my family and clients. The information in this book is not intended or implied to be a substitute for professional medical advice.

As you go through this book, you will discover and learn how your body works on the energetic level. I will explain each of the bodies in detail and explain how they work. I will also teach you how you can heal the emotional, mental, spiritual and physical body. As you learn, you will be able to help yourself, your family and your friends.

I have been working in the Healing Arts for over twenty years and now it is time for me to help you become whole again. My prayer for all of you is that through God, Jesus, Holy Spirit, The Blessed Mother, your healing team and mine, the Angels, Archangels and the Ascending Masters that you would receive in abundance all that you need through your healing. May God Bless you and your family with His special graces and His healing Love.

# Healing with Energy

Your body energy is a powerful tool and it can do many things. By accessing your energy field you can assist in healing the physical, mental, emotional and spiritual bodies as well as diseases and addictions that have been in your family genetics and generations.

There are many ways that your body can heal. Healing your body through the physical body can mean that you have an energy blockage that is preventing your body from receiving the energy that it needs to heal. Removing the blockage through energy work will allow the energy to return to that area in your body so that your body can start to heal.

There are many modalities that can be used to clear the energy blocks in the body that are very successful. For example; Energy Kinesiology, Reiki, Healing Touch, Body Alignment, Touch for Health, Massage, Acupuncture just to name a few.

Mental energy blockages in the body can be tied to a belief that is no longer serving you such as, I am not worthy.

Emotional energy blockages can be related to fears, anger, depression, anxiety, unforgiveness, trauma, stress, abuse etc. Emotional blocks are usually memories of something that happened in the past. I would say that 90% of blockages in the physical body are stuffed emotions and issues that were never dealt with.

Spiritual energy blockages can be negative energies trying to prevent you from moving forward into the Divine Light and your

Life Purpose. Here are some examples: fear of the unknown, fear of the future, anger at the past and not able to forgive someone. Spiritual blocks are usually things that are taking your peace and stopping you from connecting to God.

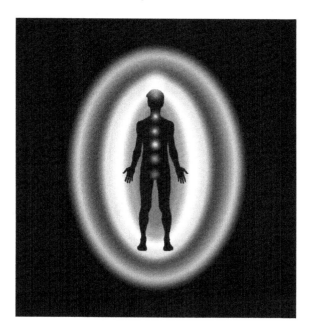

This picture shows the different layers of energy around our physical body and the energy centers of the body called the chakras. When the energy fields around our body are blocked, this can cause disease (dis-ease) in our physical body.

Removing any energy blockages in your auric field (referring to the mental, physical, emotional and spiritual energy around the physical body) will allow the healing energy from God and Mother Earth to start bringing the body back into balance so our body will start to heal. Our body is designed to heal. Our job is to listen to what our body is telling us. Our body is designed with everything it needs to heal, we just have to LISTEN. As we clear out the energy blockages and toxins getting ourselves back

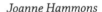

into balance, our physical body will start to heal. Now we are on our way to our true authentic selves. First we are going to learn about the physical body and how it works on the energetic level and what has helps me heal the physical body.

# *Physical Body*

Your physical body is made up of bones, muscles, organs, cells, systems, glands, tissues along with many more parts. Your body works together as one very smart system. If one part of the body becomes weak or damaged, your body will find a way to compensate to keep you as healthy as it can. You have to give the body what it needs to heal. This could be energy work, Prayer and meditation, healthy foods, supplements, essential oils, exercise, cleanses or detoxing just to name a few choices.

So what stops the body from healing? I have discovered that 90% of energy blockages in the physical body are emotional. What I mean by this is that we have stuffed our emotions, hurts, traumas, anger, unforgiveness, fears, childhood pain, abuse and anxiety into our physical body. These emotions usually go to the weakest part of the body or to specific organs. When this happens you have created an energy block that is in or around your body in the energy fields. This block will not allow the healing energy that is needed to penetrate until it is removed. The energy coming from God –Universe and Mother-earth into your body will not be able to help you because of these blockages. The energy will go around the blockages. When this happens that part of the body gets weaker creating disease (dis-ease) in the body.

Here is an example. You start to get a pain or stiffness in your knee. At first you ignore it hoping that it will go away. Then you notice it is hurting a bit more, so now you use Icy Hot or take an Advil for relief. This stage goes on for a while until this doesn't work anymore. So now it's time to go to the Doctor for x-rays, cortisone shots, surgery etc. Now I am going to tell you what I would do. When the pain first started in my knee this is a warning signal from my body that something is not right. Your body will always give you a signal, it is your job to listen to your body and get the help it needs to heal.

Knees have to do with stubbornness, inflexibility and fear of moving forward. I would figure out what is happening in my life that I am resisting. This could be change at work, not wanting to do something that would cause change for fear of the outcome.

Fear is really about trying to control the outcome. If we move forward into the unknown we know longer have control of the situation. We think change is bad and I am fine staying here even if it makes me miserable.

Once you acknowledge the situation it takes 5 minutes to release the blockage so your body can heal this. It is that simple. The key is to listen to the warning signs of the body and release the cause. I will teach you how to release the emotion as you continue to read.

# Where does this energy come from?

This healing energy is universal and is around and inside of us. It comes from connecting and breathing in God-Universal energy through your God cord which is located at the top of your head and Mother Earth energy by connecting your feet to her core and breathing it up into the body. This energy connects to the chakras.

The chakras are the energy centers in our body in which energy flows through. There are seven chakras in the body. There are also chakras above and below the body but we are just going to focus on the 7 chakras of the body.

Are body needs this energy to stay healthy. This energy is our life force. How our body gets sick is that we have energy blockages in our energy fields that prevent this energy that we need to heal. Most of these blocks in our body's energy fields are emotional. Emotions energy blocks that we have stuffed into our body because it was to painful for us to deal with. This would include childhood pain, traumas, lost, betrayal, abandonment, abuse etc. Most addictions are people trying to numb the pain caused by holding on to a secret of something that has happened to them or something that they did. All the drugs, alcohol, sex, gambling, shopping, etc will not fill that void or stop the pain. It will help momentarily but it will not go away until the pain or secret has been released and removed from the energy field.

## The 7 Chakras of the body

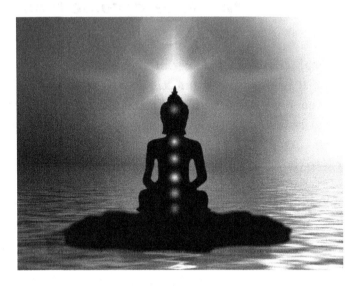

- <u>Root</u> –Base of the spine. Represents our foundation and grounding. Color is red. Eat red foods to heal this part of the body such as berries, beets, red cabbage, cherries, cranberries, watermelon, tomatoes, peppers, etc. Eating the color that corresponds with that part of the body supports the chakra energy healing. So if you are having trouble with your legs, knees, feet. Eat red. If this chakra is out of balance the effects relate to issues of physical security affecting your thoughts and feelings.
- <u>Sacral</u>- Lower abdomen. Located below the naval. Represents abundance, well-being, sexuality. Color is orange. Eat orange foods to support healing in this area such as oranges, peaches, apricots, squash, carrots, cantaloupe, sweet potatoes, pumpkin, etc. If this chakra is out of balance the effects are craving of physical pleasures and addictions. Examples are food, drink, sex, thrill seeking, exercise, appearance, sleeping pattern behaviors and worry or stress.

- <u>Solar Plexus</u>-slightly above the navel. Represents self-worth, communication, confidence, personal power and will. Color is yellow. Eat lemons, zucchini, pineapple, mangos, bananas, corn, peppers, etc. This will help support the digestive system. The effects of being out of balance are thoughts and feelings of power. Desire to control and being out of control. Feeling over powered by others.

- <u>Heart</u>- Center of the chest. Represents our ability to Love. Color is green. Eat foods such as kale, spinach, greens, green beans, etc. This will help support the heart and blood. The effects of being out of balance are relationship problems, forgiveness of self and others, fears around giving and receiving.

- <u>Throat</u>- Base of throat. Represents our ability to express how we feel in truth and love. Color is blue. Eat blueberries, eggplant, blackberries, etc. This will help support the thyroid, throat area. The effects of being out of balance are poor communication. Not able to speak ones truth.

- <u>Brow</u>- Third eye in the middle of the forehead. Represents intuition and wisdom. Color is indigo blue. Eat foods that are dark blue like berries. This will help supports the brain. The effect of being out of balance is keeping your third eye closed because of fear. How do you feel about spirit?

- <u>Crown </u>– Top of head. Spiritual connection. Color is purple. This is your connection to source. Support this with prayer and constant union with God, Jesus, Blessed Mother, Holy Spirit and the Angelic realm. Drinking water is very important in moving energy. The effect of being out of balance is your thoughts and feelings about God and spirituality.

# The 12 Major Meridians of the Body

Another way energy flows in our bodies is through meridians. Meridians are the energy arteries of the body. These energy channels transport life energy through the body. They are invisible but they bring vital and balancing energy to all systems of the body. There are 12 major meridians in the body.

Major Meridians of the Body

- Lung
- Large Intestine
- Spleen
- Stomach
- Heart
- Small
- Bladder
- Kidneys
- Circulation/Sex
- Triple Warmer
- Liver
- Gallbladder

These major meridians of the body are responsible for nourishing their corresponding organs fueling and feeding them with this life force energy. Energy flow will affect how we feel, think and our health.

As you get older all of your hurts, fears, sadness etc. will continue to go to the weakest part of your body or a specific organ until one day you go to the doctor and he finds damage or disease in your body. It's like a hurting knee or back that continually gets worse no matter what you do. What has happened is that the energy block in your body has stopped the healing energy from getting to that part of the body so it can't heal. The result is disease or damage. Our body is designed to heal. We just have to listen to our body and give it what it needs. This is very simple. Clear the energy blockages and toxins out of the body so that the healing energy can get to that place in your body to heal.

I am going to show you about how emotions affect specific organs in your body and share with you some important information to help you. Then we are going to clear the blockages in your body by doing the healing mediation. You can use this meditation as many times as you need it. With God, Jesus, the Holy Spirit, your I Am presents and Divine healing team they will know exactly how to help you.

# Emotions can Affect Organs

Specific emotions are held on to by our body parts. Let's talk about stress. Stress is very hard on your body because you are constantly holding on to it. That takes energy. Stress affects women and men differently. Men hold stress in their heart while women hold stress in their reproductive system and nervous system. To much stress for a long period of time can lead to a heart attack in men and female problems in women. Why? Because every time a stressful situation comes your way, it creates a bigger, more dense energy block in the body which stops the healing energy from getting to that part of the body. The key is not to let it in the body. Find a way to release stress. Examples; Walking in nature, biking, swimming, yoga, breathing exercises, running, taking a bath. Find healthy ways to relieve stress.

## Stress Release Technique

Here is a very simple way to let go of stress. Place your hand on your forehead and take a couple of deep breathes and relax. Next, visualize that stressful situation like you are a fly on the wall. Watch the situation like you are watching a movie with no emotional attachment to it. When you are done, take your hand off your forehead and your stress will be gone. If you feel that the stress hasn't completely cleared, do it again. The key is to watch with no emotional attachment, just watch it. At the end see the situation healed and you are happy. Always have a positive ending.

The reason this technique works is that in the middle of your forehead directly above the eyes you have two Emotional Stress Release points (called ESR points). By placing your hand on your forehead, you activate these points to release stress in your body which helps to calm you down. Parents do this automatically when their child is hurt or crying. You hold your child and place your hand on their forehead not realizing that you have activated their ESR points. The result is they calm down.

You can use this technique for any situation in life. For example, if you have a fear of flying. The night before you fly, place your hand on your forehead and close your eyes. Imagine yourself getting ready for your trip. Visualize that it is a beautiful day. Then see yourself leaving your house and going to the airport feeling wonderful. Next imagine walking through the airport and boarding the plane. Visualize the entire experience as positive. See yourself getting on the plane, you feel good. The plane takes off and then lands at your destination. Lastly, watch yourself walking off the plane feeling wonderful. What you just did was tell your brain that when you fly everything is fine. This technique takes the emotional charge out of the body. The reason that this works is because the brain doesn't know if it is real or imagined. So because you went through the situation and you saw and felt it as positive the fear leaves and your body says, I have already done this and it was fine.

You can use this technique for any stressful situation such as giving a speech, talking to your boss, planning your wedding or preparing for a job interview. It works really well for kids who are afraid of going to school or riding the bus. Kids will respond instantly to this technique.

Perhaps your child is having trouble at school. This could be writing, reading, classmates or even separation anxiety. Ask them to give the anxiety a number, 10 meaning a lot of anxiety and 0 meaning it's gone. Place your right hand on your child's forehead and the left hand at the base of the skull. By covering the forehead with your hand the points will be activated. Talk your child through a visualization technique with your hand on the forehead. For example, have your child see what is stressing (him/her) out by just looking at it with no emotion. Then have them create a wonderful day at school. See them reading, playing and having fun doing whatever seems difficult. Tell them to visualize that it is a beautiful day and all the kids are so kind and happy. Make it a wonderful day. At the end make sure your child sees himself happy. Now ask them to give the anxiety in their body a number. If the number is not 0 do it again. The next day they will feel at peace about going to school. By accessing the ESR points the brain told the body that everything is fine.

## **Healing Meditation**

This will also help release blockages in the body caused by a situation or an emotion such as stress, fear, overwhelmed, anger, unforgiveness, untrusting, etc. I would suggest that you find a quiet, peaceful place. You can even add some relaxing music as you do this. Read thru this procedure so that you have an idea of how it works. I also have this guided meditation on CD that can be purchased in the back of the book. First, let's bring in the Light.

Beginning Prayer;

> Father-Mother God, Holy Spirit, Jesus, my healing team, Angels, Archangels, Ascending Masters and anyone else of the Light that I need, I call upon you to send the Light for my perfect protect and my Highest good and I ask that what is lifted at this time that it would be replaced with something of greater value.

Whatever it is that you are feeling, allow yourself to feel it. Now get into a quiet comfortable position and close your eyes. Imagine that Jesus and you are walking into a lagoon of purple water. When the water is at your waist submerge yourself into the water as Jesus waits for you. In the water, Archangel Michael and Archangel Raphael are waiting to help you. They are going to hold you in the purple water. Allow this water to flow thru you. Now take a deep breath and allow your body to feel where this situation or emotional block is in your body. The block will feel heavy, or tight. Whatever you are feeling in your body, give it a shape.

It could feel like a knife in your back or heart, a heavy wooden cross or a big backpack on your shoulders. Maybe it feels like a heavy rock or a tight bandage around your chest. You might have shackles on your wrists and ankles trying to hold you back, there might be a bag over your head trying to be invisible and dark glasses not wanting to see the truth, a rope or brace on your neck stopping you from speaking your truth, black pants on your legs stopping you from moving forward. Maybe cement boots not allowing you to move forward in your life, etc.

Whatever shape you give the pain or pressure it doesn't matter. Just take it off or maybe you need to cut it off with a scissors. Use whatever you need to get it off.

If you are having a hard time with getting it off, just ask the angels for help and they will remove it for you. Keep handing it over to Archangel Michael or just throw it into the water. After that area is clear. Go to the next block.

Take a deep breath. Is there something else that needs to be released? Feel it and give it a shape and get rid of it. As you are going thru this process the water might turn a deep purple. Just continue removing things from your body.

Continue this process until you feel the relief. Before you leave the purple water make sure that your body feels light and your pain is gone. As you remove these blockages, you might feel heat or cold as your body releases. You might feel tingling in your body. That is the energy coming back in because the blockage has been removed.

When you feel that all discomforts are gone, jump out of the water feeling so free and happy. Jump into Jesus' arms and let him fill you with his unconditional love. This is a pink light that will embrace you. When you have been filled with all the love that you need, walk with Jesus to the shore and a beautiful angel will put a white robe with a color light inside the robe on you.

The color inside could be purple- divine love, gold- the highest color of healing energy from God, green- healing, Pink-unconditional love, blue- peace and calming or it could be a combination of many colors. Whatever color you get is fine. They know what they are doing. This robe will help to protect you while your body heals.

At this point you will be feeling GREAT! Now say, I am (your name) here and now. This brings you back into your physical body. Now we are going to integrate this healing into your physical body. See yourself in present time taking that beautiful you with the robe on into your arms. Now just love yourself. Tell yourself what a wonderful, kind and loving person you are and that Jesus will always be with you and will always protect you.

When you with the robe is filled up with enough love, you will integrate into yourself bringing all that healing into your present body and you will have the robe on. It's like your healed self with the robe on melts into you in present time. Now just ask your healing team to integrate and lock in all of this healing into your body and say, I am (your name) here and now and tap twice on the top of your head. This brings your body back into present time and integrates. While you are saying the ending prayer cup your ears with your hands to lock this healing into the body. To cup your ears place your thumb on the bottom by your ear lobes and your pinky finger over the top of the ear with your fingers behind your ears on the skull. Hold these points while saying this prayer.

Ending prayer:

> May the Light of the Divine surround me.
> May the Love of the Divine enfold me.
> The Wisdom of the Divine speak through me.
> The Power of the Divine protect me.
> The Presence of the Divine watch over me and may Unconditional Love emanate from me. Amen I thank you Father-Mother God, Holy Spirit, Jesus and everyone of the Light for your help in this healing.

Now tap twice on the top of your head to seal it.

## **Wasn't that Amazing! It is that simple.**

You can do this Healing Mediation to remove any energetic blockages in the body. This was given to Sr. Dorothy and I from Jesus and is very powerful. It is called Energy Kinesiology. I have worked with this for over 20 years with my colleague Sr. Dorothy Merth. We have continuously seen miracles in our lives and in are clients. This truly was a gift that was given to us and we want to share this simple but powerful Healing Mediation with all who are in need as a Blessing from God.

"Oh, Lord my God, I cried to you for help, and you healed me." Psalm 30:2

When you go into the water with Jesus you might see yourself at a different age. Your body wants to heal the Age of Cause which might be age 7. The Age of Cause is the age in which you first stuffed the emotion or event into our body. We choose to stuff it instead of dealing with it. I have taken many clients back to age 6 or 7 to heal. This seems to be a very powerful age.

The angels will always take you to the place or age that is going to clear this out of the body, so your body can heal. Stay at that age or place and feel what you're feeling don't run away. Bring Jesus into that place and ask him to heal this. He will put you in his arms and love you. After the pain is released Jesus will take you outside to play. Do what you loved to do as a child and ask Jesus to bring your child like spirit back into your body. When you have played enough and you are filled with joy Jesus is going to integrate that child into your present time body. It will feel like the child just melted into your heart and all that healing and joy will come back to you. That little child has now been healed and all the healing is integrating into present time.

You can use the Stress Release and/or the Healing Meditation to clear any blockages in any part of the body. The Stress Release is a quick and easy way to remove stress. For a deeper healing, do the Healing Mediation.

When you are in the water you might see cords on you attached to your chakras or around your body, just remove them. These are cords of fear and control that other people have attached to you. You don't need them so pull them off or ask Archangel Michael to take them and to heal and seal those places with light and love. When you are around a person and you get a stomach ache it is because the person has attached to you. Just close your eyes and pull out the cord, sending it back to them in love. Then put yourself in a purple bubble of light as protection. The cord might be around your neck because they are trying to stifle you, do the same thing. Pull off the cord, send it back to them as love and put yourself in a bubble of purple light or white light.

Sometimes you are around a person and when they leave, you are exhausted. Same thing cut the cords. Some people will unload their emotional garbage on you and connect to you for your energy. Always pay attention to how you feel around certain people. Are they feeding you energetically and you feel lifted or are they draining you and you feel worst? If you have people that drain you of your energy learn to protect yourself when they are around. Put yourself in a bubble of purple light and put mirrors on the outside of the bubble to reflect their negative energy back to them. Be with people who feed you spiritually and energetically.

You might also be taken to a past life or experience during your healing mediation. Your body will take you back to where you need to go to clear the cause of the blockage. It will go to where and when it first started. Wherever you are taken it's ok. Heal from that place. You can't do anything wrong. Remember God is always watching over you and He loves you unconditionally and so does your Healing team and Angels. They will guide you and help you to feel the emotions. As you feel them and acknowledge what is going on it clears that fast. You don't have to worry about anything just relax and let go and let God.

If your pain is not releasing ask yourself out loud, "What is the payoff for this pain? Some people will keep their pain because they don't want to move forward, they don't want to get a job, fear of change, fear of losing something like money, whatever it might be, let it go. Release it into the light and trust God. He will help you. You are not alone.

# *Organs that hold emotions*

Our body organs and parts will absorb specific emotional energies. I am going to help you to understand what energies affect certain organs and what can help to support the organ so it can heal. Let's start with the liver. The information in this book is not intended or implied to be a substitute for Professional Medical advice. Always ask your physician if it would be ok for you to do.

## Liver

The liver holds onto anger. Living or working in a situation where there is constant complaining, negativity, frustration, guilt, rage, or inner struggle is not good. The liver is very important to the body and is the largest internal organ. Also, it is the body's principal organ used to detoxify all the impurities that find its way into the body before entering the circulatory system. The liver is located in the upper right quadrant of the abdomen below the diaphragm. Sometimes you can feel sharp pains in this area of the body. Listen to the warning signs of your body because your body is trying to help you.

I am going to share what has worked for me. Always check with your physician.

I would first do the Healing Mediation to release the anger block in the liver. Then I would do a simple cleanse.

To help cleanse the liver, this tea is simple but effective.

*To flush the liver use 2 tsp of either fennel, anise, or fenugreek seeds with 1-2 cups of water and drink as a tea. You can do this flush first thing in the morning and then wait 15 minutes before eating breakfast. It is best to do this flush for three to seven days.*

*Another option to consider is go to your local health food store and get a Liver Cleanse. The best time to cleanse the liver is during the Spring Equinox but you can do this anytime.*

I have also used this to cleanse the liver and the gallbladder together.

## **Apple juice flush**

*Drink 1- 2cups of Organic apple juice every hour (14 cups total per day) for two days. Drink nothing else but water.*

*At the end of the second day, drink ½ cup of olive oil and ½ cup organic orange juice mixed together before bed. Lay on your right side for at least 30 minutes when you go to bed.*

*In the morning mix 2 tsp sea salts and 4 cups of warm water and drink. Make sure that you are close to a bathroom for a couple of hours. That day just eat light. The following day you will feel amazing. I like this cleanse because it is short and you get results fast. Make sure you eat light for at least 24 hours.*

## Gallbladder

The gallbladder holds onto anxiety. The gallbladder is a small pear-shaped muscular sack that acts as a storage tank for bile. The gallbladder is located behind the liver on the right side of the rib cage. The pain from the gallbladder is caused when a gallstone or stones get stuck in the duct that carries the bile from the gallbladder to the intestines. This blockage in the duct can cause nausea, bloating, vomiting, pain in the stomach, shoulders, middle of the back and middle of the chest. There are many ways to clear the gallbladder and dissolve the stones. You can use a Tincture from the health food store or Amazon. There are many recipes on the internet or by using the book The Ancient Cookfire by Carrie L'Esperance which I highly recommend. She has many very powerful methods to clear stones. You can also find a Juicing Recipe to clear gallstones.

When I had gallstones I juiced 3 times a day an apple, 2 carrots, 1 beet root and a handful of blueberries for 7 days and drank water all day. You can eat light meals but stay away from greasy foods. My stones were gone in two weeks. To keep my body clean I drink one of these drinks daily first thing in the morning. Eating apples and drinking lemon water every day is a simple way to keep your organs clean. Remember to always consult your physician before any of these remedies.

## Apple Cider Vinegar drink

*I drink 2 tsp of Braggs Apple cider vinegar, "with the mother" about 1/8 tsp of baking soda mixed in a 8oz glass of water. This keeps your body alkaline so that it can heal faster. If you can't do Baking soda just drink the vinegar and water.*

## Master Cleanse

*1-2 cups pure water*
*1 fresh squeezed organic lemon*
*1/8 tsp cayenne pepper or as much as you can handle*
*1-2 Tbsp real maple syrup (grade B)*

*Drink this first thing in the morning and don't eat for at least 15 minutes. You can also do this wonderful cleanse and shed unwanted pounds by drinking this all day for a couple of days. When I do this, I drink about 4-6 glasses a day for about 3 days. Your body feels so energized by doing this.*

## The benefits of the Master Cleanse

- Dissolves congestion in all body parts.
- Cleanses the digestive system and kidneys.
- Helps purify cells and glands in the body.
- Helps joints and muscles be more flexible.
- Relieves pressure in the nerves, arteries and blood vessels.
- Flushes the body of toxins.
- Helps heal ulcers in the stomach.

The reason that this helps heal ulcers is the cayenne pepper kills the bacteria called H. pylori that is causing the ulcer. I drank this for 7 days every morning, first thing and by the 2nd day my pain was gone. My ulcers have never returned.

## Kidneys

The kidneys hold fears, disappointments, and failures. The kidneys are located on both sides of the spinal column mid-back just below the rib cage. They are about the size of your fists and are shaped like a bean. The kidneys filter about 120-150 quarts of blood everyday to produce 1 to 2 quarts of urine and wastes along with extra fluids not needed by the body. Lemon water is a great way to keep the kidneys clean. You can also imagine blue light surrounding the kidneys. Color vibration is very powerful to the body. You can look at colors, imagine them around the organs, place colors on the spot that needs healing. If you are having kidney problems, ask yourself, what am I fearing?

Fear of:

- The unknown
- The future
- The past
- Being criticized
- Being alone
- Abandonment
- Anger
- Being blamed
- Bondage
- Not having what you want
- Not being cared for
- Children
- Competition
- Being controlled
- Darkness
- Dark forces
- Being depended on
- Depression
- Destruction
- Being dominated
- Being dumped
- Failure
- Freedom
- God
- Not being healthy
- Being humiliated
- Hunger
- Hurt
- Ignored
- Being inadequate
- Not being accepted
- Water

- Women
- Men
- Intimacy
- Authority
- Sex
- Confined
- Not being able to breathe
- Rejection
- People
- New situations
- Violence
- Making decisions
- Loneliness
- Pain
- Left behind
- Being persecuted
- Picked on
- Losing face

Use the Healing meditation to clear these fears from the kidneys and then surround the kidneys with blue light.

To detoxifying the kidneys you can use the Chinese Wolfberry. This has been used for centuries as a kidney tonic and detoxifier. You can also use the Essential oils Helichrysum with juniper or fennel. Place 1-3 drops of the oils in water and apply as a compress over the kidneys for 20 minutes. Remember to always consult your Doctor to make sure it is good for you to do.

## To strengthen the kidneys drink

8 ounces spring water
¼ cup cranberry juice
½ lemon juice

## Adrenal Glands

When we are stressed the adrenal glands release our fight or flight hormones called adrenaline and cortisone. This increases your heart rate and breathing. The adrenal glands are part of the Endocrine system. The adrenal glands release over 50 different hormones that influence many functions in the body from your energy level, mental focus, libido and your stress level. They are located above the kidneys and secrete a number of different hormones like corticosteroids which are metabolized by enzymes either within the gland or in other parts of the body.

Many people are stressed all the time and are causing a condition called Adrenal Fatigue. This happens to healers and people working in the energy fields of other people.

There are many factors that are causing Adrenal Fatigue;

- Diet and nutrition - to many processed foods, sugars and preservatives.
- Sleep Deprivation-not able to stop the brain and relax.
- Alcohol
- Stress
- Working to many hours on electrical devices.

## Symptoms that your adrenals are fatigued;

- Chronic fatigue - tired all the time
- Decrease in sex drive
- Low blood pressure
- Mood changes
- Headaches
- Abdominal pain
- Muscle weakness

- Salt cravings
- Not sleeping
- Loss of appetite
- Weight loss

**To help your body recover take;**

- B - Complex Vitamins-these B vitamins help reduce adrenal fatigue by helping the breakdown of food into proper energy so you have more energy and cell metabolism.
- Vitamin C – It's one of the most important nutrients to our immune system and is needed for the production of all your adrenal hormones.
- Magnesium – Deficiency of magnesium often results in fatigue, depression, muscle cramps and insomnia.
- Ashwagandha and Holy Basil – Improves energy levels and mitochondrial health, normalization of blood glucose, blood pressure, helps with stress.

There are many Adrenal Formulas in capsules that can help you.

Here are a few:

- Liquid Active Adrenal
- Megafood Adrenal strength
- Unlimited Heath Adrenal Relief
- Christopher's Adrenal Formula
- Soloray Adrenal Caps

Remember to always consult your Doctor. The essential oils such as Nutmeg, Sage, Clove, Rosemary, or Basil can help to support the adrenal glands.

## <u>Lungs</u>

The lungs holds on to grief, sadness and/or hurt, which represents not being able to breathe in the joys of life. Pneumonia is an emotional wound that has never healed. Bronchitis is an inflamed environment. When you experience breathing problems you are not allowing yourself to breathe in the joy of life. Remember to always take deep breaths into your stomach not your chest.

The function of the lungs is to transport oxygen from the atmosphere into the bloodstream, and to release carbon dioxide from the bloodstream into the air. Essential oils such as Eucalyptus can be helpful in opening up the head and lungs if you have congestion. Place a couple of drops of Eucalyptus oil in hot water and make a steam bath and breathe it into your lungs.

You can also use a diffuser. A diffuser is a device that you can use distilled water only and essential oils to make a fine aromatic mist that will provide distribution of the oils for hours. You can use your diffuser with different blends of oils to bring peace and calming to your home or work place, to help you sleep, to remove stress. There are all kinds of different blends that can be very helpful.

To open the lungs, rub up and down the middle of your chest with your fingers starting at the base of your throat to the middle of your chest. This technique signals the lungs to open up so it will be easier to expel the mucous. The Healing Meditation is very powerful to release blocks in the chest area. When doing the meditation allow your body to feel that pain and cry it out. You may feel a huge rock on your chest, take it off and throw it into the water. It might feel like a cable wrapped around your diaphragm cut it off. It might even feel like a straight jacket wrapped around you. Whatever it is take it off and throw it in the water or give it to Archangel Michael. When you are finished with the healing meditation take a deep breath and you will feel lighter and you will be able to take a deep breath.

## Heart

The heart is the center of love and security. The arteries carry the blood which represents the joy of life. This is why it is so important to connect with people in love. I often see older people in nursing homes losing the joy of life because they have lost their connection with their loved ones. They long for a hug from their children and grandkids.

Our hearts need love to heal. Love is the most important vibration. Jesus healed with love and love alone. Heart problems come from blocking the energy around the heart. This can be stress, closing your heart to love because it doesn't feel safe anymore to love because of a hurtful situation, unforgiveness, anger, abuse or fears. Issues around the heart can be very uncomfortable and it's hard to talk about things that **have** hurt you. The things that have hurt you is the key. These people and situations are in the past. Don't let them control your future. If you don't let them go you are bringing them into your future and why do you want to hold on to the pain.

Panic attacks and anxiety are also issues of the heart. Anxiety occurs when you feel that your life is out of control or you can't control the situation. This makes you feel vulnerable and not safe. When panic attacks or anxiety occurs you start to breath short breathe only in the upper part of your body like you can't get enough air.

To stop this, close your eyes, put your finger tip in the space between your nose and upper lip and breathe into your ***stomach*** through your nose so the energy is going through your body and exhale through your mouth and ask Jesus to take this and fill you with his peace. Keep breathing slowly into the stomach through your nose and exhale out your month. Do this for a few minutes and your symptoms will go away. If it doesn't go away I would call your doctor.

When doing the Healing Meditation with matters of the heart Jesus and the Blessed Mother are always with you and will help you. When you go into the purple water with Jesus you might become the age you were at when this happened. That is fine.

Ask Jesus to heal you and he will. Stay in the purple water and allow it to leave. At the end Jesus will give you that child in your arms. Love that child and when you received enough love the child will integrate into your body bringing all that healing to you in present time. Don't be afraid to let it out. You might have to cry, or get angry and punch the person. However it needs to come out let it out in the purple water with Jesus. He will help you every step of the way.

People think that the void or hole in their hearts can be filled with material things, alcohol, sex, drugs and people. That void can only be filled with having a relationship with God. All the addictions only last for a time but God's love for us is eternal.

I just want to say something about our blood. Blood is our life line and it carries oxygen to our organs but it also carries joy. Joy has been lost. Joy comes from God. It's that feeling when your soul is right with God. It's that inner peace that cannot be shaken by circumstance. Even when the world around us is in chaos you can still feel God's peace inside.

**"The joy of the Lord is my strength." Words to live by.**

## Breasts

The breasts hold hurts and represents not feeling loved and appreciated or a lack of feeling nurtured. The right breast represents not being able to say no and trying to please everyone except yourself. It can also represent holding on to childhood pains, abuses or trauma as well as the need to control everything because of fears such as not letting go of an emotional hurt, betrayal and unforgiveness.

The left breast holds onto fear, rejection, disappointment, shame, guilt, needing to do everything by yourself, exhaustion, insecurity and regret. Imagine that you have surrounded your breasts in green healing energy. Sending love and appreciation to your breasts is very important because your breasts need to be nurtured. Use the Healing Mediation to remove the energy blocks. Remember that when you go into the purple water with Jesus you might be back at that situation of abuse or betrayal.

That is ok. It just wants to heal and remember you are safe, Jesus is there. Allow yourself to feel where the pain or situation is in your body. Allow it to go. The breast is close to the heart, so when you are healing your breast you might see a knife representing a hurt in your heart. Just pull it out and hand it to Jesus or Archangel Michael will take it. Then ask Jesus to heal that wound and you will feel a warm peace come over you. Continue to give the feelings a shape and throw it into the purple water. You might see a tight band around your chest, just cut it off. Maybe someone is stepping on you, remove the foot. It could be something heavy like a boulder, throw it into the water. Keep removing until you can take a deep breath and you can't feel anything left on your breasts, chest, and heart.

When you have been hurt numerous times it's hard to forgive.

It is important that after you do the meditation that you call on Jesus or the Blessed Mother to help you heal your broken heart. They will help you. Visualize that you have ½ of your heart in one hand and the other half in the other hand. Now say, "I am one in heart" three times while you are bringing your hands together. Finish with your hands together on your heart and ask Jesus or Mother Mary to heal your broken heart. You will feel a warming in your heart area for a few minutes. Just allow this energy in and open your heart to receive this healing.

## Forgiveness

I just want to talk about forgiveness for a minute. People think that by not forgiving the person that it is hurting them. This is not true. By forgiving the person who has hurt you, it is allowing you to take back your power. Forgiveness has nothing to do with the person who has hurt you, it is about freeing yourself so you can move forward.

Forgiveness is a powerful word and act. So many people are being held back in life because they are not able to forgive themselves or someone else. First, the past is gone and what happened back there is over unless you continually bring it forth into your future.

Whatever you did forgive yourself and move on and try to be a better person and don't repeat that lesson. If someone did you wrong, you don't have to accept it but you have to forgive the person in order for you to be free. Forgiveness is a part of the healing process. If you can't forgive you can't heal and if you can't heal you will not be able to move forward. By not forgiving you are only hurting yourself. Unconditional Love is a very special kind of Love. It is <u>Love without condition</u>. It's unique, it's genuine and it's real. Love heals all. Jesus said, and the greatest of these gifts is LOVE. Love everyone and everything, especially yourself.

If you need to forgive someone put them in the purple water with you and Jesus. Now say to them, " I love you, I am sorry, please forgive me and thank you." You have now released them and forgiven them. Give that person to Jesus and say, " I am taking back all of my power that I have relinquished to you and I will never relinquish my power to you or any one again. Good bye and God bless. Now put your hand on your forehead and see all the power coming back to you like white sparkling energy into your body and you are getting 6 feet tall, 8 feet tall, 10 feet tall. Now say three times," I am standing in my power and in my truth." As you say this feel how strong and powerful you really are. Then tap twice on the top of your head to lock this in.

## Throat

When you are experiencing tightness in your throat, it is because you are not speaking your truth. It could also be that someone is choking you energetically. The throat and the mouth have to do with speaking. If you are holding onto your words or anger this could create problems in the mouth and stomach. Stuffed anger in the mouth can create cold sores. Festering words or anger in the mouth can be swallowed into the stomach causing indigestion, acid reflex, stomach aches and gas.

If you can't speak your truth to this person, write it down. Just get it out of the body so that it doesn't damage the body. When you feel that you said it all. Tear up the letter.

You can burn it or bury it, but don't reread it. Give it to Jesus and ask him to fill you with his love, peace and healing energy. Ask Archangel Michael to remove the block in your throat and to surround your throat with blue light inside and outside of your throat. You will feel instant release. Use the Healing mediation to remove the energy blocks.

You can also bring that person into the purple water with you. Have Jesus stand between you and speak your truth. Give the person to Jesus and say,

**God, you are (name) helper in every way, you are his/her health and his /her wholeness.**

Now give the person to God, take a deep breath and let it go. This is a very powerful prayer of submission. If anyone asks me to pray for them I say this. The reason that it is so powerful is that you surrender that person and the situation to God and you are asking him to take care of it. I have no clue of what is going to help that person, but God knows. **When we surrender everything to God or Jesus that is when miracles happen. Let go of the control.**

## Esophagus

The esophagus is also known as the food pipe. Its function is to assist in food passing from the pharynx to the stomach. When this gets inflamed it can cause many problems. Croup in children is an inflammation of the esophagus caused energetically by an angry household or environment. Swallowing feelings of grief, anger, festering words or hurt. Staying silent by holding onto how you are feeling can also cause problems. If you need quick relief for croup go into a bathroom and turn on the hot water. The steam will open up the esophagus. If it is cold outside, the cold will also help.

Acid Reflex takes a toll on the Esophagus also. Try rubbing under your left breast using your pinky finger side of your right hand and breathing deep into your stomach. This will stop the acid production in the stomach and give you instant relief. Make sure that you are breathing deep as you rub. Why this works is because there is a point halfway under the breast that will be sore as you rub. Rubbing this specific point will also help.

Aloe Vera juice (1-2 Tbsp daily) helps relieve Acid Reflex and help support the digestive system. Aloe Vera juice can be taken in the morning and at night. By adding a Digestive enzyme and a Probiotic to your diet daily will also help. As we get older our digestive system gets depleted and needs a little help.

Digestive enzymes, Aloe Vera Juice and Probiotics can be found at any health food store. Probiotics are also found in yogurt. Make sure you eat the yogurt with the live bacteria. The Greek yogurts are good because they have more protein in them.

Here is a good drink for inflammation in the body.

*8 oz of warm or hot water*
*1 tsp real maple syrup*
*½ of an organic lemon juice*
*½ to 1 tsp Organic Turmeric spice*

*Mix together and drink like a tea. You can drink this everyday to help with inflammation in the body.*

## Mouth

Your mouth speaks your truth. If you are not able to speak your truth in love and continually have fear of expressing how you feel you could also develop cold sores around and in your mouth. Fresh organic garlic kills harmful bacteria and viruses. At the first sign of a cold sore, sore throat, running nose, or respiratory cold use garlic. Peel a clove of garlic and cut it in half, placing ½ of garlic on the inside of each side of your cheek. The garlic will mix with your saliva and enter your system. If you can't tolerate fresh garlic, use Garlic capsules, but fresh is always better. You can also use Oregano essential oil on your feet to kill viruses and bacteria in the body. This oil is very powerful so don't use it in your mouth. There are capsules that you can take that are very good also. Elderberry in any form is very good for flu or colds.

Bad breathe has to do with not letting go of anger and revenge from the past. Forgive the past, it is over and done with. When you can't forgive you stay in that pain. You are living in the past which is holding you back from your future. Let it go! Surrender it to Jesus and ask him to fill you with his peace. Say,

**I release the past, I am free, I forgive myself and everyone.**

Then ask the angles to invoke the formula of Love around this, activate the code and bring this to the highest level of consciousness. Feel it leaving your body. You will feel instant peace. By holding onto this you are only hurting yourself.

## Teeth and Gums

Teeth and gums have to do with not being able to make a decision and believe in that decision. Root canals have to do with not being able to bite into a belief that is no longer serving you. Your foundation is being shaken and having to create a new foundation that serves you. Gum Disease stems from not being able to make a sound decision. If you are having gum issues like gingivitis there is a toothpaste by Young Living that is made with Thieves essential oil that works very well. Oil pulling

37

helps remove toxins from your teeth and can also help with gum disease.

## Oil Pulling

*Use a tablespoon of coconut or sesame oil and swish the oil in your mouth for exactly 20 minutes. Discard the oil from your mouth and brush your teeth. This can be done daily as needed.*

## Jaw

Your jaw holds tension. This could be tension from not speaking your truth, anger, stress, resentment or anxiety about a situation or person. When your jaw is stressed it starts to hurt causing TMJ. What has helped me with TMJ is to rub under your collerbone on both sides with your thumb and middle finger using your right hand. While doing this open and close your mouth slowly until pain is gone.

Applying the Essential Oil peppermint on the outside of your jaw can relieve pain from your jaw.

The Healing Meditation can help here also. When you go into the purple or blue water you will be able to feel what is on your jaw and release it. It might be wired shut because you are afraid of speaking your truth. You might have a helmet on or some kind of protect that is stopping the healing energy from getting to the jaw. Take it off. Keep taking off until your jaw feels clear then rub the points under your collar bone while you are opening and closing your mouth. Your pain and tension should be gone. Heart blockages will also radiate pain or pressure in the jaw. If it doesn't go away go to the doctor and get checked out.

## Sinus

Sinus trouble has to do with someone or a situation being in your face. The sinus area holds the emotions of irritation, annoyance, and frustration with other people's behavior and not letting it go.

To help open the sinuses, rub the points in the middle of the cheeks on the cheekbones for about two minutes'. You can also rub the points in the hollows of the eye by the eye brow and continue rubbing along the brow. These points will be sore.

Using a Neti pot can be very helpful. A Neti pot can be bought at any drug store. It is a pot or a squeeze bottle that you fill up with DISTILLED WATER ONLY and Pure ionized salts. Remember to always use distilled water to avoid infection. The Neti Pot is used to rinse out the sinus cavity and is very effective. They also have saline nose sprays that are very effective.

Using a Sinus Decongestant can also relieve sinus pain. To open the sinus cavity and to get your sinus to drain, I have used the Essential oil eucalyptus in a sink of hot water. Put 3-5 drop of the oil in hot water in a sink then place a towel over your head and the water. Breathing the steam from the water will help open up the sinuses.

Using the Healing Mediation can help you talk to the person who is in your face. Remember to bring them into the purple water with Jesus between you and speak your truth.

Then give the person to Jesus and say, Jesus, you are (the person's name) helper in every way. You are her/his health and wholeness" now give the person to Jesus and take a deep breath and let it go.

Surrender all you problems and worries to Jesus. He will take the burden and help you. The key is to let it go.

**Jesus, I surrender this to you, please take care of it.**

## Allergies

When people develop allergies to things it can be emotional. I will give you an example. Say you are a child and you are at a park playing. You can smell the lilacs in the air. Now a bee stings you. Your brain remembers that when you smell lilacs you were afraid. So year after year goes by and when the lilacs are in bloom your allergies come back. You can heal this by using the Stress Release points. If you remember when your allergies started, go back there. Holding the point on your forehead see the whole situation like you are a fly on the wall just watching with no emotion. Make sure that you create a positive outcome. You have now taken the fear out and the allergy will be gone. Here is another example. Do you have allergies when you are around dogs? Ask yourself, was there a time when I was frightened by a dog? If yes, do the Stress Release. You can also do the Healing Mediation to clear allergies.

## Nose

The nose has to do with recognition of self. A constant runny nose is the inner child crying. Ask yourself as a child, why are you crying? Maybe your inner child needs to be loved. In your mind, see yourself loving your inner child. It might need to play. Play with your inner child. I think a lot of us have forgotten how to play and to have that sense of joy and wonder. It is very healing to play and to be outside in nature.

Having a bloody nose has to do with not feeling noticed. To stop a bloody nose put the **opposite arm** up like a scarecrow so that the shoulder and elbow are in alignment and the hand is pointing upwards to the sky with the palm of hand opened away from the body. Hold this pose for a minute or two and the bloody nose will stop. I have used this many times and it works every time.

## Ears

Earaches and infections in the ears have to do with not wanting to hear something. What is it that you don't want to hear? It could be anger, advice, hearing that you did something wrong or arguing in the home. Babies will close the ear energy if there is anger in the household which result in ear infections. If someone is telling you something and you don't want to hear it, you will close down the ear energy.

Warm Sweet oil in the ear can be very soothing or you can use NutriBiotic ear drops also if you feel you have an infection. Nutribiotic is a natural antibiotic made from grapefruit seed and works very well both products can be found at a Health food store or Amazon.

When using the Healing Mediation notice what is on your head and your ears. It can be ear muffs or you may even have a helmet or bags over your head trying to be invisible. If you clear the energy that is blocking your head and ears, the pain will subside and the body will start to heal. Use the Healing Meditation to clear this.

## Eyes

Eyes are like the ears. What don't you want to see? It could be chaos in the home or workplace. This could be weight gain in yourself or others, relationship problems, procrastinating work that needs to be done. I have seen many children getting glasses when their parents are getting a divorce. What happens energetically is that you put some kind of a block over your eyes.

Energetically, the block could be dark glasses, a bag over your head or a bandana over your eyes. These are blocks that are stopping you from seeing what you don't want to see.

Use the Healing Meditation to clear this. First when you are in the purple water see what is on your eyes and get rid of it in the water. Then look at what you don't want to see and then surrender the whole situation to Jesus and let him fill you with his Love. Remember to see a positive ending.

## <u>Hips</u>

Hips have to do with your balance in life. If your pain is on the right side of the body, this represents your male energy. The left side is your female energy .This can tell you a lot about what is happening in your body. If you aren't able to take in feminine energy your left side will be weak. It is about honoring and nurturing your feminine side. The right side of your body is masculine energy. Honoring your masculine side of being able to let go of situations and find strength. The tail bone has to do with your grounding into Mother Earth.

Balance in life is about your life being balanced with play time, work, rest, meditation, prayer, exercise and spending time with family and friends. When your hips start hurting, a part of your life is out of balance. Many of us are working to many hours and not enjoying our life. Ask yourself, what is off balance in my life? Be honest with yourself. Getting your life back into balance will help your hips balance. Energetically this also could be that you have closed down your solar plexus and sacral chakras which have to do with communication and relationships.

Use the Healing Mediation to remove the energy blocks in this area. This area of the body needs to be grounded into Mother Earth energy. Imagine that you are standing on earth. See that there are roots coming out of your feet going down into Mother Earth crystalline energy. Now breathe this up through your legs into your body up to the top of your head. You are now grounded. You have to be grounded to manifest your dreams.

When you are doing the Healing Meditation in the purple water your blocks could be heavy like a boulder, or constricted like a wrap. Whatever you are feeling give it a shape and throw it into the water. You might see heavy black spandex pants on your hips and legs. Just let them go.

## Knees and ankles

Legs, knees and ankles have to do with moving forward in your life. If you are experiencing any pain in the legs it has to do with moving forward in your life. What is holding you back? What are you afraid of? Any kind of change that you are afraid of will trigger this.

Do the Healing Meditation to clear this. Energetically it will look like your have bound your legs or ankles with a rope or cable. Sometimes you will have cement boots on because you are dragging your feet. If this has been going on for many years, you probably have many layers of black spandex pants on that have stopped the energy flow to the legs. There could be braces on your knees and maybe you feel a shooting pain like a knife. Just keep taking it off of you. As you clear the blockages your legs will become tingly because the energy block is now gone and the healing energy is coming in to heal this area.

There might be a wall in front of you stopping you. All you have to do is imagine that you have taken a white light sword from your heart and use the sword to knock down the wall and ask Archangel Michael to clear your path. Put your sword back into your heart. This sword is a spiritual gift from God the help you. You can use it to clear negative energy in a room or to cut cords from you.

At the end of your Healing Meditation imagine yourself moving forward with ease and excitement into a new day filled with Blessings from God. This will bring in new energy which will help support you.

## Shoulders

Shoulders hold onto overwhelming burdens. Things that you will not let go of like hurts and things from the past. Energetically this looks like a huge backpack on your back or it could be many different sacks over your shoulders or even a heavy wood cross that you are burdened with.

When you hold onto the past or the many things that you are trying to control, it not only affects your shoulders, but it affects your back and neck. Until you release those burdens and junk that you are hanging onto any kind of treatment will only be temporary. When doing the Healing Meditation, make sure you are feeling the shoulders, neck and back. If you have a huge backpack on your back it is blocking the energy to the back and spine.

Arnica is a gel that can be helpful in relieving pain and swelling.

It also helps with arthritis. Tart cherry juice is also good. I buy R.W. Knudsen juices because they have no sugar and can be found at any supermarket. Turmeric capsules are great for inflammation issues also. Olive oil is also wonderful in relieving pain and healing the joints. Add some peppermint oil to the olive oil for quick relief.

## Back and Spine

The back and spine represent your support system. Do you feel supported by life, relationships, family, or work? Financial fears are always related to lower back problems feeling like someone just stuck a knife in your lower back. Go into the purple water and pull out all that stuff in your spine. There can be tight belts, knives, arrows. Make sure that you pull out, then take a deep breath and feel again. Keep taking things out until your back is clear. Then ask God to send the golden healing light to your back.

Neck problems on the spine are related to burdens, worries and carrying baggage from the past. A lot of the time when you are in the purple water you will see a huge backpack covering the spine. This can be anger and hurts that you won't let go of. It could be your worries and fears. Maybe it is financial burdens that are weighing you down. Whatever it maybe it is covering your spine meaning you do not feel supported.

When you take this off in the purple water ask Archangel Michael to heal and strengthen your spine. You will feel a warm sensation on your spine as he brings a white-blue light to heal your spine. The curve part of the neck is very important part in connecting with the Divine. If you are having trouble with this part of the neck do the Healing Meditation and ask the angels to help you heal this part of your neck and to open the connection.

Meditation will also help but make sure you ask the angels to close and protect this spot on your neck after your meditation.

## Hands and Arms

Hands represent your ability to give and receive. The left hand is your receiving hand and your right hand is your giving hand. Make sure that you are always receiving money with your left hand not your right. The hands can get out of balance with too much giving and not equally receiving or vice versa. Mothers are very good at giving and not receiving. The arms have to do with embracing and enjoying life. Put your arms around yourself and give yourself a big hug. Allow yourself to be loved and nutured. A lot of people have been hurt and it is hard to let other people into your heart again. Start by loving yourself and ask Jesus to help you to open your heart to loving again.

The emotional cause of arthritus in the fingers is self punishing, feeling like a victim and blaming self. Ask yourself, "Why am I punishing myself?" It could be something from the past that you are not forgiving yourself for. Put your hands in purple water and pull off what is on your hands. It could be gloves with nails in them, sticks in your fingers not allowing them to bend. Whatever it is take it off and throw it in the purple water. After you are finished put on white gloves for protection. Also using olive oil on your hands at bed time with help heal the joints. The spice turmeric is also good to help with inflammation. Turmeric can be found in capsule form also.

## Digestive System

The digestive system includes the colons, large and small intestines, sigmoid colon, rectum and anus. The digestive system is all about **letting go of the problem or situation** you are carrying within you. Emotions that can affect your digestive system are hurt, anger, fear of letting go and unforgiveness.

The reason why emotions affect the digestive system is because we take in the energy of communication through our solar plexus chakra which is located by our belly button. If we feel threatened in any way we close this chakra down so nothing gets in or out. Have you ever had an argument with someone and after the argument your stomach hurts? What is happening is that either you took in that negative energy or you closed it down. If you are not able to forgive someone or a situation this will affect your digestion. It is important to keep your digestive system healing because your immune system is located in your digestive system.

This is where constipation starts. Not drinking enough water or eating enough raw vegetables and fruits will also contribute to constipation. To get your digestive system moving, release the energy block by asking yourself, what am I holding onto? Then rub the outside of your thigh starting at the knee up to your hip bone. Using your fingers inch up on the outside of your thigh up to your hips bones three times. This opens the channels to your digestive system. If you have the diarrhea, do the opposite by inching your fingers downward three times from the hips to the knee to close the channel. It is helpful to do the Healing Mediation here also because there might be cords attached to your solar plexus (navel). Sometimes people will attach to you with cords that connect you to them. This is not good. When people attach to me I can feel it instantly. Let's say that every time you are around a certain person, when you leave you don't feel well. They have just attached to you and are taking your energy. This is what I do and I also do this after every session with my clients. I imagine that I have a big beautiful sword of light in my heart. I touch my heart and the swords come into my hands. I now use the swords over my body to cut all attachments on me. This only takes a minute. Then I ask Archangel Michael to send them back in love and to heal those spaces in me.

Sometimes people will attach to you out of fear or control. You will feel better when the cords are detached. Then put the swords back into your heart. To protect myself when I am around negative people, I put myself in a **bubble of white divine light from Jesus, gold light from God and a purple light bubble. On the outside of the purple bubble I stud it with diamonds or mirrors** reflecting that energy back to them. This is very powerful and can be used anytime. Teach your children to protect themselves especially if they are sensitive to others energy.

To support the digestive system you can take Aloe Vera Juice 1-2 Tbsp daily in the morning. As we get older digestive enzymes and probiotics are also very important in supporting your immune system which is located in digestive system. The drink Kombucha is an excellent way to support the digestive system. It contains live probiotics and organics acids like vineagar. I drink this once a week to keep things moving with ease. For occasional irregularity Shaklee makes a wonderful herb product called Herb-Lax.

## Stomach

The stomach is another place where all of the emotions enter. Have you noticed getting a stomachache after an argument or diarrhea because you are afraid or fearful of a situation. Have you noticed difficulty digesting what life is throwing at you? Are you feeling like you are of being attacked? Most people gain weight especially around the middle as protect because they don't feel safe.

Stomach ulcers can be caused by negative thinking and your outlook on life. Like a situation that keeps festering. The emotions can be fear, worry, and anxiety. When you let the emotions keep festering and are not able to let it go, this can cause trouble in the stomach. Try to think of a time that you were so worried about something. Now ask yourself, was it worth all the worry? Did you worry about things that never happened. Worry is such a waste of time. Worry creates anxiety. Surrender your worries to Jesus and keep moving forward. He will take care of it. I have learned that when we worry we are not trusting God. So God sits back and says you try to fix this yourself and when you are ready to give this to me I WILL take care of it. God will not step in until you are ready to give it to him because of FREE WILL.

Once you let it go, He will send thousands of angels to help you. The key is to truly give it to God. Surrendering is trusting in God.

You can clear the energy blocks by using the Healing Mediation. Using the Master Cleanse can be helpful in healing the stomach. Cayenne pepper is one of the best spices for healing ulcers.

Remember to consult your physician to make sure that if you are on medication that you will be safe.

Drink the Master Cleanse first thing in the morning 15 minutes before eating and before bedtime for 7 days. After the first day you will be able to feel the difference.

To help clear inflammation in the Digestive system you could use:

*1 tsp of Turmeric spice and 1 cup of warm milk*

This will help with any inflammation in the colons and intestines.

49

Another way to stimulate and get the digestive muscles working again is to eat celery and blueberries between meals. This will help the muscles get back in shape and help to heal the digestive track.

## Parasites

Everyone has some form of parasites in their body. The emotion attached to parasites if you are having trouble getting rid of them is giving your power to others and letting them control your life. Parasites can be on the outside or inside of the body like Scabies. Ask yourself, Who is controlling me? Put them in the purple water with Jesus and yourself. Look to see if that person is attached to you. You might see shackles on your wrists and ankles, maybe cords wrapped around you, cords attached to your chakras or maybe even a body bag around you.

Whatever it is ask Jesus or Archangel Michael to remove it even if you don't see it they will take it. Then ask them to fill you with white light and put you and that person in separate bubbles of white light and give them to Jesus. As the person is going to Jesus take back your power. Say Jesus, I surrender (name of the person) to you. Now you say, I now take back all the power that I have given you and I will never relinquish my power to you or anyone again. See the power coming back to you as white sparkling light and see yourself getting bigger and stronger. Put your hand on your forehead and say, I stand in my power and in my truth three times. See yourself happy and free then tap twice on the top of your head.

What I do to keep myself clean of parasites is use a combination Tincture of Black Walnut, Clove and Wormwood three days before, during and after the full moon. If you can't find the combination tincture buy them separately. You can get this at any Health food store or on Amazon. Before you go to bed, take the tincture drops in one tablespoon of water.

Pumpkin seeds are also good to cleanse the body of parasites. For Dogs, you can boil a bunch of parsley and use the water in their food and water. You can also get a Parasite cleanse if you think you need a little more help.

There is a book called The Cure for all Cancers by Hulda Clark were she believes that an over load of parasites in the body and other things can produce cancers. It's a very interesting book.

Spiritual parasites can also be a problem especially if you are dealing with skin issues or restless leg syndrome. To clear spiritual parasites, ask the Gold and Silver Angels to shower you with a high vibration purple light <u>inside</u> and <u>outside</u> of your body. Close your eyes and see yourself standing in a purple shower of light. Stay in that shower until you feel peace. Then ask them to put you in a white fluffy diamond studded jump suit for protection while you heal. Continue to do this every night before you go to bed until your skin has cleared.

## Clearing Parasites

*Take Black walnut, Clove and Wormwood Tincture before bed in 1 tablespoon of water three days before the full moon, on the full moon and 3 days after the full moon. It will tell you on the bottle how many drops to take.*

<u>This works because Black Walnut and Wormwood kills the adults and the Cloves kills the egg of the parasites.</u>

## Detoxifying

It is very important to keep your body clean from pollutant in the environment, food and water. Here are some of the remedies that I use to keep my body clean.

Archangel Michael said that we need to bless our food before we eat it and say over your food. 88-88-88-88 and hum the tone G. This will change the vibration of the food to be healthier for your body. When saying the eights, its eight – eight pause, eight – eight pause, eight – eight pause, eight –eight pause, then hum the tone G.

## Apple Cider Vinegar

*Mix 2 tsp of Braggs Apple cider vinegar with 1/8 tsp Baking Soda in 8 ounces of water. Drink this first thing in the morning. This will help your body stay alkaline so your body can heal faster.*

## Epsom Salt and Clay Baths

*Any kind of bath salts like Himalayan salts with Essential oils are good.*

*Taking an Epsom salt or clay bath every month is very helpful in detoxing your body. I use 1-2 cups of Epsom salts in a bath tub of water. Soak for 20 minutes. When I am soaking, I imagine that I am in the purple water and all the toxins are coming out of my body thru my skin. You can buy Epsom salts at any store. They are very inexpensive.*

*I also use Pascalite Clay Powder from Wyoming. This is a wonderful product. I use ¼ of a cup in my bath tub. This is very good to remove heavy metals from the body. Soak for 20 minutes in the clay. When you are done and empty the water, you can see the metal flakes on the bottom of the tub.*

If you are not able to soak in a bath tub, soak your feet. I would use about ¼ of the amount that you would use in the tub and soak for 20 minutes. When using a foot massage detoxifier, be careful and don't use it to much because it can deplete you of essential minerals. Emergen-C vitamin pack that you add water to contains vitamin and minerals to replenish the body. I drink this every morning. It's simple, easy and tastes good.

## PectaSol-C

PectaSol-C is a supplement by ecoNugenics that has many benefits.

• Supports Cellular Health
• Supports a healthy Immune System
• Removes toxic Heavy Metals

This supplement is a natural product derived from the pith of citrus fruit peels, including lemons, limes, oranges, and grapefruits. I order this on-line. If you our experiencing a metal taste in your month you need this product.

Master Cleanse is very powerful. I love this cleanse and it's easy. I do this when I am starting to feel sluggish and when I have not been eating the cleanest. You feel so good after a couple of days.

## Master Cleanse

*1-2 cups pure water*
*1 fresh squeezed organic lemon*
*1/8 tsp cayenne pepper or as much as you can handle*
*1-2 Tbsp real maple syrup*

*Drink this first thing in the morning and don't eat for at least 15 minutes. You can also do a wonderful cleanse and shed unwanted pounds by drinking this all day for a couple of days. When I do this, I drink about 4-6 glasses a day for about 3 days. Your body feels so energized by doing this.*

## The benefits of the Master Cleanse

- Dissolves congestion in all body parts.
- Cleanses the digestive system and kidneys.
- Helps purify cells and glands in the body.
- Helps joints and muscles be more flexible.
- Relieves pressure in the nerves, arteries and blood vessels.
- Flushes the body of toxins.

## Himalayan salts

*Himalayan salts have many uses from cooking, clearing negative ions in the air using the lamps and using them in bath water. I place about 3 rocks with purified water in a pint glass jar with a plastic cover over the top. With a plastic spoon I drink 1 tsp of this in 8 oz glass of water every other day. This contain trace minerals needed in the body, rich in iron, balances alkaline/acidity in the body, dissolve and eliminate sediment in the body.*

# Subconscious Mind

So I bet you are wondering, "How do I know what to do and if it is good for me? " The subconscious mind holds all the information that you need. I use my intuition, Kinesiology and the pendulum to access this information.

Your intuition is that still voice inside of you. Some call it that knowing, or gut feeling. This will get stronger for you through meditation. When I started going down the path of a healer, I didn't always trust the answers that I was receiving. I am going to show you a few things that I used that are easy to learn and very effective.

If you are a Healer you probably are already working with the Pendulum. A pendulum is a tool used to pick up your energy or the persons energy that you are working on. Using your pendulum is very quick and effective. I am also going to give you a warning. The pendulum is not God. God wants you to go to him for help, not to put your trust in the pendulum. How I use the pendulum is as a verification tool. It keeps me on track with channeling so that I am not connecting to the clients stuff and not giving my opinion. It helps me to be that clear channel for God to work through. There are many classes on how to use the pendulum if you are interested.

Just remember when using the pendulum to **ask statements, not questions.**

Examples:

- **It is in my best interest and High Good** to take this vitamin.

- **It is in Lisa's best interest and Highest Good** to go for a different job.
- **It is in my best interest and Highest Good** drink cranberry juice for my bladder infection.

Let's say that you got a yes that you are to drink cranberry juice for your bladder issue.

Now you would find out how many times a day you should drink cranberry juice by saying, It is in my best interest and highest good to drink cranberry juice at least once a day, twice daily, or more. Your pendulum will give you a yes to verify .Your pendulum will stay in neutral position until you get to the right dose and then swing right meaning yes.

I use the pendulum along with my intuition to access clients and my information from the subconscious mind. The subconscious mind has all the information that you need to heal. Think of this as memory recall. Your conscious mind is awareness at present moment. Like your environment, the chair that you are sitting in, and your breathing. Learning to master the pendulum can be difficult because you can't connect at all to the answer or outcome. Remember you are the clear channel that God is working through. See yourself as the extension cord that is connecting God and to the person you are helping. This has nothing to do with you so don't connect with it. Let it flow.

Another way to access information from the body is Kinesiology. Kinesiology is the practice of muscle testing. Muscle testing is very easy also. Have the person raise their arm up straight until it is even with their shoulder. Tell them to hold it straight and strong.

First you have to make sure that they are not switched. If there energy polarity is switched you will not get correct answers. With their arm in position ask or say to their body, Give me a yes. Now push their arm gently downward. If this is a true statement to their body, the arm will show resistance and stay strong. Now say, give me a no. The arm will weaken. If when you say to the body, give me a yes and you get a weak response the polarity is switched.

To correct: use your hand to go up and down the middle body starting at the pubic bone to under the nose up and down several times. Keep your hand in front of the center of the body about 3 inches away from the body. **Make sure you stop at the nose.** This is called Flushing the meridian. With the clients arm in position say, give me a yes. You will now get a strong arm meaning that this is a true statement to the body. Then say, give me a no. The arm should go weak. It is going weak because it is not a true statement to the body. Now you are ready to access to subconscious mind.

Ask them to state their name, my name is Joanne. You will get a strong muscle test because that is a true statement to their body. Now ask them to say a different name, my name is Bob. Then test their arm and there will be weakness. They will not be able to hold their arm strong because this is not a true statement to their body. It works like a lie detector test. Your arm will stay strong if this is true to your body. The arm will go weak if it is not a true statement to your body.

When I am at the Health food store and I want to know quickly if I need this vitamin, this is what I do. You are going to use your body. This is so simple. Make sure you are standing straight and tall. Check yourself by saying body give me a yes. Your body will move forward and no, your body will move backward. You will actually feel your body moving forward and backward. Then take the vitamin or whatever you want to test to see if your body needs it and place it on your navel. Then say it is in my best interest and Highest Good to take this vitamin. Your body will move forward meaning yes it is good for you and your body needs this. No, your body will move backwards meaning you don't need it. You can do this anywhere.

Your body or I AM presences has all the information that it needs to heal. You just need to listen to what your body is telling you.

Prayer and mediation is the most powerful way to connect with your I AM presence, God, Jesus, your angels, healing team, etc.

"Be still and know that I Am God" this is so true. You will not be able to connect unless you quiet your mind, turn everything off, take some deep breaths and **listen.**

# The Mental Body

We've covered the physical, emotional body and now we are going to talk about the mental body. The mental energy body is like the knowing. It gives you the ability to think thoughts, have beliefs, discernment along with higher psychic abilities. Let's talk about beliefs. Beliefs can be generational and even genetic. There are so many people that belief that they are not worthy. This will affect your life in a big way.

Let's break this down. I am not worthy of what..........

- Love
- Money
- Forgiveness
- Promotion
- Blessings from God
- Soul Mate
- Joy
- Happiness
- Health
- Abundance of everything I need
- Family
- Children

So when you believe that you are not worthy, what happens in your life?

- Abandonment
- Poverty
- Not able to move forward from hurt
- Promotions pass by you

- Lack of miracles
- Loneliness
- Sadness
- Depression
- Sickness
- Lack
- Dysfunction
- Separation
- Anxiety

I see this all the time in my practice, people feeling so discouraged and trying to change their lives and nothing is working. They will say to me that they feel stuck.

The reason this is happening is because locked in the sub-conscious mind and cell memory is the belief sabotaging their life.

So you can believe that you are worthy but if your cell memory and sub-conscious mind believes differently nothing will change.

There are many beliefs that we have created for ourselves but there are also many beliefs that are passed down from the generations.

I will give you a few. I am not...

- safe
- loved
- healthy
- whole
- forgiven
- at peace
- moving forward with ease

- trusting in life's processes
- feeling safe to grow up
- responsible for my actions
- choosing to live my life now
- caring for myself or others
- loved or wanted
- open to new ideas
- joyful and grateful
- adequate at all times
- forgiving myself or others

So many people live in fear. They are so fearful of things that will never happen. It is as though they create all this negativity around them because it feels safe. Fearful people need to be in control of everything around them and everyone. As long as they feel that they are in control they fell that they are safe. But they are not. They are so fearful of change because they can't control it. So what happens is they stop all the blessings from God because they can't control the outcome.

Here are some examples of fears...

- Fear of not being accepted – so you don't go to the party.
- Fear of authority – so you won't ask for a raise or stick up of yourself.
- Fear of failure – so you don't even try.
- Fear of being blamed – so you won't speak your truth.
- Fear of God – you think God would never forgive you.
- Fear of rejection – I am not going to be hurt again.
- Fear of being inadequate – why try and look stupid.
- Fear of change – I might not like it and I am fine.
- Fear of intimacy – I am not going to get hurt again.
- Fear of new situations – I might not be safe.
- Fear of moving forward – I can't control this.

There are so many fears in our lives that are controlling us and we don't know why.

It is because they are stuck in are cell memories and subconscious mind. So how can we clear this? I am going to give you a short but powerful healing modality that has helped me.

We are going to start with healing fear, because everyone has some form of fear in their lives.

Be in a quiet place and close your eyes. Now just breathe and connect to Mother Earth's beautiful energy and breathe it into your body to the top of your head. Then connect your God cord into that beautiful Golden healing sun of God and bring it into the top of your head and down to your toes. Call in your healing team and angels and anyone of the Light that can assist you in this healing.

Now say," I know how to live without fear"

If you are testing this statement your body would move backwards because you don't believe this. It is not truth to your body. If you use a pendulum you would get a negative spin.

Now say, I invoke the formula of Love around this. The formula of love is Gods transforming divine energy of love for you.

Now say," Activate the code." This is a special healing code that will clear this for you. Everybody has a special code that only the subconscious mind knows and your healing team will invoke this.

Then ask the Angels to bring this to its Highest Level of consciousness.

You will actually feel this coming out of the body. When you are done you will feel Gods peace and love surrounding you.

You can use this process to clear beliefs that are stuck in the cell memory and quantum field. Here are a few affirmations that you can use.

## Positive affirmations

Emotion | Affirmation
--- | ---
Fear | I know how to live without fear.
Hurt | I am free.
Anxiety | I welcome joy and ease into my life.
Anger | I care for myself and others.
Guilt | I release the past. I am free. I forgive myself
Self rejection | I accept myself.
Rejection | I am perfect and loved.
Self hatred | I am full of joy and self love.
Loss of power | The world and I are safe.
Insecurity | I am free to speak up for myself.
Inflexible | I am open to all ideas.
Burdened | There is time and space for all that I do.
Confusion | My mind is relaxed and at peace.
Grief | I gentle follow with life.
Resistance | I fill my world with joy.
Family friction | I am loved and wanted.
Untrusting | I trust in life's processes. I am safe.
Tension | I trust life. I am safe.
No direction | I move forward with ease.
Judgment | My feelings are normal and safe.
Stubbornness | All in my life is changing.
Denial | I rejoice in all that I am.
Failure | I am adequate at all times.

| | |
|---|---|
| Over mothering | I am free to be me. |
| Feeling trapped | I move through life with ease. |
| Selfishness | I create a joyful world in which to live. |
| Humiliation | I move beyond all limitations. |
| Isolation | I am one with all. |
| Childhood pain | I forgive my parents/ everyone etc. |
| Overprotection | It is safe for me to grow up. |
| Scatteredness | I am centered. I center myself. |
| Revenge | I am at peace. |
| Narrowminded | I am completely opened. |
| Defeatism | I choose to live my life now. |
| Lost | I am whole. |
| Unhealthy | I claim perfect health and wellness. |
| Depression | It is safe for me to be me. |

Continue to use this. When I am in a healing session we can clear 5-6 affirmations at one time. I wouldn't do more because the body needs time to processes this information. Wait about a week and then clear some more. Drink water before and after healings because water helps move the energy in the body. You can also do an Epsom salt bath to help remove the leftover junk.

As you clear the beliefs that are holding your back, you will start to feel the peace and ease in your body. Things will become easier and you will no longer react to things that don't matter. When you are at peace in your mind and body that is when miracles happen. Why? You are now trusting God! This is such a beautiful place to be in. Every day I say ten times, Jesus, I surrender this to you, please take care of it. I give him my day and all my worries for the Glory of God. Then I say, **The Best Is Yet To Come!** This will bring in hope.

# Choose Wisely

We all have the ability to choose if we want to be happy or sad. When you are sad, do something that brings you joy. You can change how you feel by the thoughts that you choose. You can change the emotions that you are feeling by staying out of someone's chaotic life. YOU HAVE THE CHOSE TO CHOOSE HOW YOU FEEL. It's called FREEWILL and it was given to you by God. People always say, I FEEL........ So instead of FEELING SAD, change it and FEEL HAPPY. Remember you are in control of how you FEEL. Say I AM JOYFUL. I AM HAPPY. I AM HEALED. I AM PEACEFUL.

I always say, **"Don't let other people take your JOY."** Remember misery likes company. Not in my world! I refuse to go down that road. If someone is having a bad day try to help them see the glass half full instead of half empty. If that doesn't work send them love and ask Jesus to help them see the truth in the situation. Then REMOVE YOURSELF and let Jesus work. It's not your lesson so don't take it on.

Some people will try to push your buttons to get you angry because they had a bad day. Don't respond. If you respond in anger to try to defend yourself all of their baggage has now been dumped on you. Now you feel angry and they feel great. Your anger opened the door for them to dump their junk on you.

Here is an example;

Your spouse comes home after a rough day at work. You are sitting down and watching a show. You are happy, relaxed and at peace watching your show. Now he says, Must be rough just sitting there when you could be cleaning. He just pushed your button and you become angry and say," I just sat down for 2 minutes before I start supper." This is called trying to defend yourself. At this point all his emotional baggage that he brought home has now been lifted from him and on to you. Now he goes upstairs to change and comes down so happy and refreshed and you are now in anger at what he said and on top of that you have all his junk on you. I see this all the time.

Now I am going to show you how to stop this. You can do this technique with anyone who is dumping on you. When someone is carrying to much emotional pain they try to get rid of it instead of dealing with it. All they need is a reaction from you and it is gone. When someone is trying to push your buttons or make you angry in anyway immediately imagine a purple wall of protection around you. This wall will not let it get through to you. The other thing is not to defend yourself in anger. Defend yourself in love. You know who you are and why you do the things that you do and you don't have to defend yourself for taking a break. Just say ok and walk away. If you have to explain something just speak your truth in love. You could say, Yes, I could be cleaning but I needed a break. The key is not to react negatively. This works every time. Now you still have your peace and they need to find a way to release their emotional pain. Maybe they can go outside for a walk or work out for a while.

Some people like to play the victim and they are good at it because they are getting the attention that they need. No more problems, no more attention. What they don't understand is that this is negative attention which keeps them from moving forward. I always ask my clients, what is the pay off for you to hold on to this situation? This is a very powerful statement. I will give you an example.

A client came into my office with chronic pain in her back and legs. She had been to doctors and chiropractors with no relief. When I started working on her the emotion was fear of moving forward. I asked her what was going on and she explained that she didn't like what she was doing but was afraid of the future. I asked her to give her pain a shape and a voice and ask it why it was here. She started crying and said it is keeping her from returning to the job she hated. By acknowledging her truth, her pain left immediately. We worked on moving forward in her life and her pain never returned. What was her pay off for the pain? Not wanted to go back to a job that she hated. So her body created the pain (blockage) which stopped her from going to work.

When I was going thru a rough patch in my life a wise soul (my girlfriend) said to me, "It's like going around the same mountain over and over again until that mountain has such a deep groove in it that you can't see yourself anymore." This was so true! We get stuck in our pain and we don't know how to get out of it. We keep thinking the same thoughts and doing the same things with no results.

**Choose your thoughts wisely because your thoughts create your reality.**

If you are always focusing on worry, fear and anxiety, you are bringing that INTO YOUR FUTURE. What I have learned is that you have to change the story. If you are sick, see yourself healthy and say," I claim perfect health and wellness." Put pictures of yourself around the house when you were healthy and happy. If you are going thru depression say," The joy of the Lord is my strength." See yourself filled with joy doing something you love.

When I feel sad, I always bake something. I bake because I know that by making my family cookies, it is going to bring them joy and that makes me happy. Another thing I do is go outside. I love to work in the garden. I will not allow myself to go deeper into that negative emotion. The more you concentrate on how unhappy you are, the deeper you will go into that depression. You have to stop it immediately, give it to Jesus and ask him to take it and fill you with His peace. Then do something that brings you happiness and joy. Here are some examples of things you can do.

## Things you can do

- Go outside and see the glory of God's creation.
- Cook something fun.
- Watch your favorite movie.
- Call a friend and see a movie.
- Help someone in need.
- Make blankets for the homeless.
- Visit the elderly and help them.
- Volunteer at the food shelf.
- Babysit for someone in need.
- Work at the church.
- Take a walk.
- Read books that are positive.
- Clean out a draw or closet.
- Plant flowers.
- Get a dog.
- Bring joy to someone else.
- Do the Healing Mediation

When you are not focusing on yourself and helping someone else you immediately feel the joy.

Remember you are in control of how you feel and how long you are going to stay in that negative emotion. It used to take me a long time before I surrender to Jesus. Then I realized that my worry wasn't doing anyone any good especially me. Now I give it to Jesus immediately. My life is more at peace knowing that Jesus has my back and I trust in his mercy and love for me.

Guard your heart at all times and don't let chaos control your life. Choose peace. Peace in your heart will bring your closer to God and your life will flow with ease. Don't sweat the small stuff because it doesn't matter. If you have dishes in your sink at night and your kids want to play. Play with your kids and leave the dishes. It doesn't matter if your kitchen is messy. Make a memory and fill up on happiness and joy with your kids or whomever.

To all the healers who are reading this book, not everyone wants to heal. You can bring a horse to water but you can't make them drink. Sr. Dorothy my teacher told me the healing is between God and the person on the table. She said the role of the healer is to be the conduit between God and the person. It is up to that person on the table to receive as much as they can from God through you. You are in that room to hold the space of love for that person. When the client's session is done and they leave your office your work is done and now the Holy Spirit takes over to help that person. Shower yourself in purple rays and disconnect any cords with your sword. If you have taken any junk from the session send it to the Universe to transmute it and send it back to the person as love.

**Let go of the outcome because it isn't about you or your success as a Healer.**

You are the Light for that person's enlightenment. What an honor to work in people's energy field. Don't take this for granted. Be grateful for your gifts and help as many people as you can for the Glory of God.

# The Spiritual Body

The spiritual energy is your bodies life force energy. It is that gut feeling that we all feel. Some people call this the soul or I Am presence. The spiritual body is a massive network of highly intelligent energy. We could not exist on earth without this energy. The spiritual body is connected to our physical body through our solar plexus chakra tucked under our ribs cage in the center of our body by the heart. This is called the Heart of Hearts and this is where I connect when I am praying or meditating. This is our connection to Source.

If you are going through some health issues this is the place to be. Your body has all the information that it needs to heal. The key is to access this information.

Jesus said, "Be still and know that I am God."

When you are still and listening to the voice in your Heart of Hearts you will receive the information that you need for your life.

When you are having work done by a person in the field of the Healing Arts this is where they work. We are the conduit between you and God. To be a Healer is such a profound gift and it takes a lot of hard work and study every day. I pray the rosary every morning and connect to God, The Holy Spirit, Jesus, Blessed Mother, Archangel Michael and his team for protection and many more. I am telling you this because it is important that people bring God back into their lives and their healings.

I found an easy way to connect to this place. Take 3 deep breathes into your nose and out your mouth with your eyes closed and relax. On the third breath in before you release that breath pause. That is known as the space between. Let that breath go but say in that space. When I am here it feels like I am laying on a cloud completely supported by the universal God energy. In this space is where you can access all the information that you need. Just breathe and let your mind empty out.

At first it might take some practice but don't give up you will soon master this.

You have to be still and stay in the NOW – present time to connect with Source energy. This is a very powerful place and don't give up, keep practicing and you will get there.

God will always give you the answer. If you aren't hearing it he will find a way for you to get it. When I first started doing this I couldn't hear anything. But I always got my answers and guidance through dreams, songs, people talking and me overhearing the conversation. Your angels will always help you get your answer and they will not stop until you get it. I also use the Bible for clarity. I would pick up the Bible and open it randomly and start reading. I would always be on the right page that would help me.

God is so good to us and he is trying to help us all the time. He loves us so much that he gave us Jesus. Jesus loves us so much that he died for us. God also gave us the Holy Spirit to be our counselor and the Archangels and Angels to help and protect us. The Blessed Mother loves us so much that she said yes to God so that Jesus could show us how to live in love. We are not alone ever! Remember we have to choose because of freewill whether or not we will accept the help.

Every morning I call in everybody to help, guide and protect me.

I surrender my family to Jesus and ask the Holy Spirit to keep them on their path and to protect them.

If you are worried about something or someone give it to Jesus and send the whole situation love and light. If we continue to worry or feel anxiety about someone or a situation we haven't let it go. God will not interfere if we won't give it up. Let go and let God and then watch God do his miracles for you!

# *Praying*

I t's very important to learn to pray. Prayer is talking to God or Jesus as if He is your best friend sitting next to you in the car. Tell him everything. Your struggles, worries, dreams and what you need help changing in your life. Jesus loves you so much and he just wants a relationship with you. We are all sinners, but he loves us so much that He died for us! What a sacrifice he endured for us because of His LOVE for US! This is Amazing Grace.

God also gave us the Holy Spirit to live in us to guide and counsel us. When Jesus went back to the Father the Holy Spirit came. Ask for the Holy Spirit to guide you and counsel you. The Holy Spirit was given to us as a gift from God.

The Blessed Mother Mary was given to us to protect us and the earth. I ask the Blessed Mother to protect my children because she was a mother to Jesus and understands. When I need something I ask the Blessed Mother to intercede for me to Jesus. Jesus never refuses his mothers requests. I pray the rosary every morning. The Rosary is a string of beads in which you pray the Hail Mary, Our Father and Glory Be repetitively. There is a website called Mary TV that prays the rosary from Medjugorje where the Blessed Mother still appears and gives us messages on the 2nd and 25th of every month. This is a great resource. Denis and Cathy pray the rosary twice a day and I pray with them on the website. Jesus said when two people come together in prayer, **Miracles** happen. Praying the rosary every day will change your life and your family. The Blessed Mother asks us to pray for the souls in purgatory, to pray for peace and the conversion of souls.

Turn off the radio and all the electronic devices and be still. Take a walk in nature and connect to that earth energy. Close your eyes and feel that energy, smell the fresh air, hear the birds. I have seen many healings happen just by being in nature. Nature brings peace and when the body is at peace the body can heal.

We have also forgotten how to connect with God even though God is all around us. Our Guardian Angels were giving to us at birth to help us and guide us. There are millions of angels sitting around because no one is asking them for help. Because of freewill we have to ask the angels for help. I have a very busy life and if it wasn't for Gods help and the Angels I would not be able to do this work and keep my life in balance.

If you need surgery don't put your trust in the doctors, put your trust in God. Ask Him to guide the surgeons so you can have the most benevolent outcome to your surgery and recovery. If you have picked a doctor and something inside doesn't feel right, find another one. This is your inner guidance helping you, listen to it.

**Whatever you do, ask for help. God will send you everything that you need. Just trust in God's mercy and love for you.**

Another piece of advice that is so important to hear is, if you are going thru a health crisis don't focus on the crisis. Immediately give it to God and don't claim it. Focus on creating your future. Plan what you are going to do in the summer months. See yourself planting a garden or taking a vacation. So many people that have been diagnosed with cancer or any illness, give the Illness the power by focusing on the diagnosis. Don't create that reality for yourself. Claim perfect health and wellness and see yourself healthy and strong. Put pictures around the house of happy times and you looking and feeling great! Create your reality. What you are focusing on, you are creating. So focus on your dreams. Don't bring fear into your future. Instead bring happiness, joy, health, love, wholeness, freedom, abundance, and peace. Be the Change! Every morning say, I claim perfect health and wellness. You can also find healing scripture and say them. Take charge of your life and do some research on your illness and find out what your body needs to heal. Change your diet and go outside to connect with the healing energies in mother earth. Be still and listen to that small voice inside and let it guide you.

# *Prayers*

Another powerful way to pray is through prayer, fasting and novenas. A Novena is an ancient devotion that consists of 9 days of prayer for a special intention. When I need something special I go to the rosary and the novena prayers. I will list a few of my favorite prayers.

## The Rosary

There are many books on how to pray the rosary. If you go to the website www.marytv.com and listen to the daily rosary with Denis and Cathy you will learn very easily.

*These four prayers are part of the Rosary.*

This is said on the Cross in the beginning of the rosary.

## Apostles Creed

I believe in God, the Father almighty, creator of heaven and earth, and in Jesus Christ, his only son, our Lord. Who was conceived by the Holy Spirit and born of the Virgin Mary; suffered under Pontius Pilate, was crucified, died and was buried. He descended into hell; the third day He rose again from the dead; He ascended into heaven, and is seated at the right hand of God the Father Almighty; from thence He shall come again to judge the living and the dead and his kingdom will have no end. I believe in the Holy Spirit, the Holy Catholic church, the communion of Saints, the forgiveness of sins, the resurrection of the body, and life everlasting. Amen

The Our Father is said on the first bead of every decade.

## Our Father

Our Father, who art in heaven, hallowed be thy name. Thy kingdom come, thy will be done on earth as it is in heaven. Give us this day our daily bread, and forgive us our trespasses, as we forgive those who trespass against us. And lead us not into temptation but deliver us from evil. Amen

The Hail Mary is said on all beads after the Our Father.

## Hail Mary

Hail Mary, full of grace, the Lord is with thee. Blessed art thou among women, and blessed is the fruit of thy womb Jesus. Holy Mary Mother of God, pray for us sinners, now and at the hour of our death. Amen

The Glory be is said between the decades.

## Glory Be

Glory Be to the Father and to the Son and to the Holy Spirit. As it was in the beginning, is now and ever shall be, world without end. Amen

After the Glory Be the Blessed Mother of Fatima told the three children to say, "Oh my Jesus, forgive us our sins, save us from the fires of hell. Lead all souls to heaven, especially those most in need of your mercy."

Pray the Rosary for the Blessed Mothers intentions of the conversion of souls to her son Jesus, for Peace, and for the souls in purgatory.

This next prayer is a very powerful prayer. The reason that it is so powerful is because you are surrendering the person to God and asking him to intercede for this person. Let go and let God.

### Prayer of Submission

*God, You are (the person's name) helper in every way. You are (her/his) health and wholeness.*

*I have seen many miracles with this prayer. The key is to completely surrender the person or situation to God. Let his will be done not yours.*

### Serenity prayer

The serenity pray is so powerful because you are accepting. It is what it is and you are not resisting or fighting it anymore.

*Lord God, grant me the serenity to accept the things I cannot change; courage to change the things I can; and the wisdom to know the difference.*

### Memorare

You can say the Memorare as a novena. A novena is praying this prayer 9 times in a row for 9 days to obtain special graces from

Jesus and for intercessions from Mary or the saints for help. Novenas are very powerful. Here is my favorite one.

> *Remember, O most gracious Virgin Mary, that never was it known, that anyone who fled to thy protection, implored thy help, or sought thine intercession was left unaided. Inspired by this confidence, I fly unto thee, O Virgin of virgins, my mother; to thee do I come, before thee I stand, sinful and sorrowful. O Mother of the Word Incarnate, despise not my petitions, but in thy mercy hear and answer me. Amen*

Remember prayer is talking to God. It doesn't have to be special prays. Pray from your heart and talk to God, Jesus, and the Blessed Mother. Get to know them and feel their love for you.

**"As the Father has loved me, so have I loved you. Now remain in my love." John 15:9**

# Confessing our sins

Confessing our sins to a priest is a very powerful freeing of the soul. If you don't believe in going to a priest to confess your sins then go to Jesus and have a heart to heart with him and let go of all the pain that you are carrying. So many people are carrying secrets from years ago. God already knows what you did or didn't do. Ask for forgiveness and release it to Him. If you need to tell someone that you are sorry, do it. If you need to ask someone for forgiveness, do it. Stop wasting time. All these secrets and baggage from the past are holding you back from this beautiful life and gifts that God has in store for you and your family.

If the person is no longer with us, write them a letter and burn or bury it. Just get it out of your body so that your body can heal. If you are not able to talk to the person you can do this exercise.

Visualize putting yourself in the purple water with Jesus. Now bring in the person that you need to say sorry to. Now ask Jesus to cut all cords of fear and control between both of you and put both of you in bubbles of white light but not touching. Now say:

I love you
I am sorry
Please forgive me as I forgive you
Thank you

This is a form of forgiveness which sets both of you free. Now give that person to Jesus and take a deep breath and release. When we can't forgive someone it's like drinking poisen and wishing the other person would die. But it's not affecting them at all. It's affecting your life and your health. Let it go and let God take care of it. Don't let the person or situation control you any longer. Set yourself free and close that door of the past behind you and know that today is the first day of the rest of your life and make it a great day!

If you are feeling guilty about something that you did in your past it's time to let it go.

Tell God that you are sorry of your sins. Any prayer that tells God you are sorry, that you will mend your ways, and that you firmly intend to avoid what leads to sin is a good Act of Contrition. When you say this pray really say it from your heart.

## Act of Contrition prayer

O my God, I am sorry for my sins because I have offended you. I know I should love you above all things. Help me to do penance, to do better and to avoid anything that might lead me to sin. Amen

## Penance

**Penance is an expression of repentance for having done wrong.**

When you go to confession the priest will give you a penance which is usually to say some prayers like, 5 Hail Mary's and 5 Our Fathers. But you can do penance for your sins by helping the sick, serve food to the poor, work at the shelters, visit the home bound or maybe help someone in need financially. Do something from the heart that will tell God that you are sorry and glorify his name through your work.

This is a very important step in the healing process. Love yourself enough to do this, you will not be disappointed.

# Spiritual Warfare

The other thing I would like to share with you is Spiritual Warfare.

I think humanity has forgotten that there is a devil and a hell. We have made up our own rules as we go through this thing called life. Reading and studying your Bible is so important in living your life. Use scripture to help you. If you are new to this watch the movie, The War Room by Alex and Stephen Kendrick. This movie will show you how to use scripture in your life. I love this movie. You can also download the scripture used in the movie from your computer.

> "Be strong in the Lord and in the power of His might. Put on the whole armor of God, that you may be able to stand against the wiles of the devil. For we do not wrestle against flesh and blood, but against principalities, against powers, against the rulers of the darkness of this age, against hosts of wickedness in the heavenly places.' Ephesians 6:10-12

David Jeremiah says in his book, The Spiritual Warfare. Satan's war against us is organized and strategic. The word principalities refers to his clever plans, crafty deceptions, and cunning methods.

Satan is trying his hardest to destroy the family and marriage bond. Pray to the Blessed Mother for protection on your family everyday. Pray prayers of protection over your family, home, cars, workplace, schools, community and world.

# God's Armory

*Stand therefore, having girded your waist with truth, having put on the breastplate of righteousness, and having shod your feet with the preparation of the gospel of peace; above all, taking the shield of faith with which you will be able to quench all the fiery darts of the wicked one. And take the helmet of salvation, and the sword of the Spirit, which is the word of God.* Ephesians 6:14-17

The books written by Stormie Omartian called,"The Power of the Praying Wife and The Power of the Praying Parent" are wonderful prayer books to help your family. She uses scripture with prayer which is very powerful.

There are scriptures to heal you, to protect you, to show you how to live and walk in this world.

Dodie Osteen has written a beautiful book on how to use scripture when you need healing. It is called, Healed of Cancer.

David Jeremiah has written a book on Spiritual Warfare with scripture to protect you.

Stormie Omartian has written books on The Power of the praying parent using scripture.

As a Healer I come in contact with many different energies. This is what I do to protect myself and you should also protect yourself when you are working in someone's energy.

Put the Armory of God on you. This scripture is very powerful. Ephesians 6:14-17

It is very important to ground yourself into the crystalline energy of Mother Earth. See your feet have roots that are connecting to Mother earth's energy 5 miles down and 5 miles across. Pull this energy up by breathing it into your body up your legs to the top of your head. Now connect to God's energy by imagining that you are connecting your God cord into that beautiful energy of a bright ball of light and breath that energy down into your body down to your feet. Now see that golden cord that is going through your body expand from the inside of your body outward to form a Gold tube of light 20 feet around you. Ask the Angels to pull in your Aura to 18 inches from your body. This will protect you. Keep reinforcing this all day.

Another protection is the Violet Flame. Ask St. Germaine to engulf you in the Violet flame 20 feet around you in all directions.

I have also used the triple protection of white light, purple light and then gold light on the outside and stud it with mirrors.

Always protect yourself or you will get sick from other peoples energy. Remember to always shower yourself in the purple rays and disconnect any cords with your swords after every healing session.

On the internet you can download, The Catholic Warrior. These are spiritual warfare prayers that can help you, your family and your clients if you are a healer. Here is one prayer that I use.

## Binding evil spirits

In the name of the Lord Jesus Christ of Nazareth, by the power of the cross, his blood and his resurrection, I bind you Satan, the spirits, powers and forces of darkness, the nether world, and the evil forces of nature.

I take authority over all curses, hexes, demonic activity and spells directed against me, my family, marriages, my relationships, ministry, endeavors, finances, and the work of my hands, and I break them by the power and authority of the risen Lord Jesus Christ. I stand with the power of the Lord God Almighty to bind all demonic interaction, interplay and communications between spirits sent against me and my family, and send them directly to Jesus Christ for him to deal with as he wills.

I ask forgiveness for and renounce all negative inner vows that I have made with the enemy and ask that Jesus Christ release me from these vows and from any bondage they may have held in me or my family. I claim the shed blood of Jesus Christ, the Son of the living God, over every aspect of my life for my protection. Amen

This is a good prayer to use if you have been in a bar or around a negative person. Remember negative energies do attach to you so keep yourself clean. I also say," This is not my stuff and I now release it and send it into the light to transmuted into love and send to humanity as healing energy."

I also carry my rosary with me and wear a crystal and metals around my neck.

It is also a good practice to sage your house weekly and use Himalayan salt lamps in your house to clear the air.

Remember that your house is open to many people and not all of them have good intentions. So keep your home a place of love, fun and healing for your family.

Here is a pray that I use to clean my house. You can use this prayer after you have a gathering at your home to clear any energy that people left in your home. The prayer is from the book Awaken To The Healer Within by Rich Work with Ann Marie Groth.

## **Prayer to clean your home**

Archangel Michael please stand at the head of my property and Archangel Raphael please stand at the foot. I ask that you would sweep my property with your golden wings and remove all entities, negative energies, physic parasites and bugs, remove all lost souls, close all vortexes and wormholes with sacred geometry and seal them. Remove everything that is not of the light and take it and dispose of it as you will. Fill my house with God's golden light of protect and healing. Thank you

The angels will give you different colors for different things.

- Gold is the highest vibration of white light from God.
- Green is healing energy usually from Archangel Raphael.
- Purple is Divine Love from God.
- Pink is unconditional Love usually from Jesus.
- Blue is peace and calming usually from Mother Mary.

Color vibration is very powerful and very healing to the body. If you know that someone is struggling ask the angels to put them in a bubble of pink light which is unconditional love from Jesus to help them. If your kids are nervous about something, put them in a bubble of blue light which will bring them peace and calming energy. If someone needs healing put them in a bubble of golden light from God or green light.

# *Essential oils*

Essential oils are some of the most powerful therapeutic agents known to man. These oils have be used and named in the Bible for healing and anointing.

I also use Essential oils from Young Living for help in healing and also for protection as I work. I love White Angelica, Sacred Mountain, Frankincense, Spikenard and Raven-sara, just to name a few. You can use these oils on the body, in bath water or bath salts or diffuse them in a diffuser. Any essential oils that are therapeutic grade and 100% pure are fine. Using Essential oils can help with many different things.

Don't be afraid to use the essential oils. Young Living has put out a PDR on how to use them and what oil will help your problem. I use it all the time and love it. You can also go to their website for products and information.

Another resource that I use is a book called, Releasing Emotional Patterns with Essential Oils by Carolyn L. Mein. This is a great reference book which is very easy to understand.

During flu season I diffuse Thieves to kill airborne viruses and bacteria.

Pepperment oil is great in relieving pain on the body.

Lavender helps with calming the body down and leg cramping.

Eucalyptus is good to open the sinus and lungs by inhaling the oil in a diffuser or steam bath.

There are many oils that can be beneficial in supporting the body in the healing processes. There are oils for anxiety, sadness, skin rashes, illness, protection, skin problems, sleep issue and many more. Whatever the problem might be you will be able to find an oil that will help you.

# Rocks and crystals

You can use crystals and rocks also on you and in your home. Here are a few that I use and love.

**Black Tourmaline** clears negative energies. I keep one in my pocket and two at the front door of my home. It can be used on your third eye for 20 minutes to help it open up more.

**Amethyst** helps alleviate migraines and nervous tension. Also improves concentration.

**Crystals** are great in every room. I have crystals hanging from every ceiling light to clear negative energies for peaceful sleep. Remember when you place a crystal in your home or wear one make sure you program it with your intention for that crystal like I did in to the bedrooms to clear negative energies for a peaceful night sleep.

**Obsidian** is also one of my favorites. This stone helps alleviate pain, reduce tension, release energies, improves circulation to speed up the healing process in wounds, help with anxiety and traumas. Keep this stone in your pocket on the side of the body that needs healing.

**Rose Quartz** helps to heal the heart chakra and keep the heart open for love. If you work on computer this stone help protect you against damaging radiation. Place the rock between you and your computer or wear a necklace. Every week clean the stone under water for a few minutes. This stone can also stimulate circulation and increase sexuality and fertility.

**Labradorite** is very effective in alleviating bone problems, disorders of the spinal column and joint problems. Put labradorite under your mattress to help you heal as you sleep.

**Agate** is used to alleviate skin problems, dizziness, headaches, tired eyes and can help with fevers when placed on the heart chakra.

**Coral** can help women in menopause prevent against osteoporosis. It is also beneficial in the treatment of blood and circulation disorders.

**Aquamarine** can be worn around the neck to treat neck and throat problems. Placing it on swollen glands will reduce the swelling. Very beneficial is treating thyroid problems.

**Aragonite** promotes good bone formation, strengthens the immune system, help reduce hypersensitivity and calcium deficiencies. Place under your pillow to prevent against nightmares and sleepwalking. Keeps the body stay calm when dealing with difficult people.

**Azurite** promotes and speeds up the healing of wounds in the body. This stone activates the liver to increase detoxing in the body and helps with sound decision making.

**Brazilianite** is a very rare and powerful healing stone. It is used to help disorders of the nervous system, brain and spinal cord. It has been very effective in the treatment of inflammations and multiple sclerosis. It strengthens the nerves and helps the body work in harmony.

**Calcite** is good for itching and inflamed skin. Calcite powder mixed with petroleum jelly and applied to the skin is very beneficial.

**Celestite** helps regulate monthly periods and relieves anxiety.

**Chaorite** strengthens courage and self confidence. Its physical properties absorb ultra-violet and x-rays so that the skin is protected. Doctors and nurses working with x-rays should wear this rock for protection.

**Citrine** its benefits the nervous system and stimulates the metabolic processes of the liver, stomach, duodenum and pancreas. It's very good for children who are having focus issues.

**Lapis Lazuli** helps promotes clear understanding and intuition. It is very effect against depression and issues relating to the head.

Always remember to clean your stones and crystals. You can wash them under water, put them outside when there is a full moon or put them in sea salts over night. This will recharge the energy in the stones and crystals. There are many different stones that you can use for many things. Find a stone that can help you.

I use the book Healing Crystals and Gemstones by Dr. Flora Peschek-Bohmer and Gisela Schreiber. The book contains pictures of the stones and crystals with a description of the healing properties.

You can put rocks and crystals in your pockets, in every room of your home, in your office and outside your home. Rocks and crystal can help you on many different levels so use them to help you and your family.

# *Quick Reference*

## *Healing Mediation and Remedies*

I put the Healing Meditation and the remedies together for quick reference. The Healing Mediation is available on CD at the back of the book.

### Healing Meditation

This will help release blockages in the body caused by a situation or an emotion such as stress, fear, overwhelmed, anger, unforgiveness, untrusting, etc. I would suggest that you find a quiet, peaceful place. You can even add some relaxing music as you do this. Read thru this procedure so that you have an idea of how it works. First let's bring in the Light.

Beginning Prayer;

> Father-Mother God, Holy Spirit Jesus, my healing team, and your healing team, Angels, Archangels, Ascending Masters and anyone else of the Light that is needed for this healing we call upon you to send the Light for our perfect protect and for our Highest good and we ask that what is lifted at this time would be replaced with a blessing.

Whatever it is that you are feeling, feel it. Now get into a quiet comfortable position and close your eyes. Imagine that Jesus and you are walking into a lagoon of purple water. When the water is at your waist submerge yourself into the water as Jesus waits for you. In the water, Archangel Michael and Archangel

Raphael are waiting to help you. They are going to hold you in the purple water. Allow this water to flow thru you. Now take a deep breath and allow your body to feel where this situation or emotion is in your body.

Is there heaviness, tightness, pain, etc. Give the feeling a shape. It could feel like a knife in your back or heart, a heavy wooden cross or a big backpack on your shoulders. Maybe it feels like a heavy rock or a tight bandage on your chest.

You might have shackles on your wrists and ankles trying to hold you back, there might be a bag over your head trying to be invisible and dark glasses not wanting to see the truth, a rope or brace on your neck stopping you from speaking your truth, black pants on your legs stopping you from moving forward. Maybe cement boots not allowing you to move forward in your life, etc.

Whatever shape you give the pain or pressure it doesn't matter. Just take it off or maybe you need to cut it off with a scissors. Use whatever you need to get it off. If you are having a hard time with getting it off, just ask the angels for help and they will remove it for you. Keep handing it over to Archangel Michael or just throw it into the water.

Take a deep breath. Is there something else that needs to be released? Feel it and give it a shape and get rid of it. As you are going thru this process the water might turn a deep purple. Just continue removing things from your body.

Continue this process until you feel the relief. Before you leave the purple water make sure that your body feels light and your pain is gone. As you remove these blockages, you might feel heat or cold as your body releases. You might feel tingling in your body. That is the energy coming back in because the blockage has been removed.

When you feel that all discomforts are gone, jump out of the water feeling so free and happy. Jump into Jesus' arms and let him fill you with his unconditional love. This is a pink light that will embrace you. When you have been filled with all the love that you need, walk with Jesus to the shore and a beautiful angel will put a white robe with a color light inside the robe on you.

The color inside could be purple-Divine Love, gold-the highest color of healing energy from God, green-healing, pink-unconditional love, blue-peace and calming or it could be a combination of many colors. Whatever color you get is fine. They know what they are doing. This robe will help to protect you while your body heals. If you can't see it that's ok they will put the protection on you.

At this point you will be feeling GREAT! Now say, I am (your name) here and now. This brings you back into your physical body. See yourself taking that beautiful you with the robe at whatever age you see yourself is fine and put (her /him) into your arms. Now just love yourself. Tell yourself what a wonderful, kind and loving person you are. When the you with the robe has filled up with enough love, you will integrate into yourself bringing all that healing into your present body and you will have the robe on.

Now just ask your healing team to integrate all of this healing into your body and say, I am (your name) here and now and tap twice on the top of your head. This brings your body back into present time and integrates.

Ending prayer:

We thank you Father-Mother God, Holy Spirit, Jesus and everyone of the Light. We thank you for your help in this healing.

When you are in the meditation just trust that they are helping you in whatever way they can and allow this healing. You can do this for just about everything from stress, to pain, to fears, anxiety, anger, depression, grief, moving forward, and moving forward in your spiritual journey.

You can order the CD which is so much easier to sit or lay down and listen to the guided mediation. Either way will work for you.

# *Remedies*

### **To help cleanse the liver, this tea is simple but effective.**

### **Tea**

To flush the liver use 2 tsp of either fennel, anise, or fenugreek seeds with 1-2 cups of water and drink as a tea. You can do this flush first thing in the morning and then wait 15 minutes before eating breakfast. It is best to do this flush for three to seven days. Another option to consider is go to your local health food store and get a Liver Cleanse. The best time to cleanse the liver is during the Spring Equinox but you can do this anytime.

I have also used this to cleanse the liver and the gallbladder together.

# Apple juice flush

Drink 1- 2cups of Organic apple juice every hour (14 cups total per day) for two days. Drink nothing else but water.

At the end of the second day, drink ½ cup of olive oil and ½ cup organic orange juice mixed together before bed. Lay on your right side for at least 30 minutes when you go to bed.

In the morning mix 2 tsp sea salts and 4 cups of warm water and drink. Make sure that you are close to a bathroom for a couple of hours. That day just eat light. The following day you will feel amazing. I like this cleanse because it is short and you get results fast.

## Master Cleanse

1-2 cups pure water
1 fresh squeezed organic lemon
1/8 tsp cayenne pepper or as much as you can handle
1-2 Tbsp real maple syrup

Drink this first thing in the morning and don't eat for at least 15 minutes. You can also do a wonderful cleanse and shed unwanted pounds by drinking this all day for a couple of days. When I do this, I drink about 4-6 glasses a day for about 3 days. Your body feels so energized by doing this.

## The benefits of the Master Cleanse

- Dissolves congestion in all body parts.
- Cleanses the digestive system and kidneys.
- Helps purify cells and glands in the body.
- Helps joints and muscles be more flexible.

- Relieves pressure in the nerves, arteries and blood vessels.
- Flushes the body of toxins.
- Helps heal ulcers in the stomach.

The reason that this helps heal ulcers is the cayenne pepper kills the bacteria that is causing the ulcer. I drank this for 7 days every morning, first thing and by the 7th days my pain was gone.

## Use this drink to bring your body into an alkaline state.

2 tsp of Braggs Apple cider vinegar, "with the mother" 1/8 tsp of baking soda mixed in a 8oz glass of water.

This keeps your body alkaline so that it can heal faster. You can do this first thing in the morning or throughout the day.

## Oil Pulling

Use a tablespoon of coconut or sesame oil and swish the oil in your month for exactly 20 minutes. Discard the oil from your mouth and brush your teeth. This can be done daily as needed. This helps remove toxins from your teeth and gums.

## Acid Reflex

Aloe Vera juice (1-2 Tbsp daily) helps relieve Acid Reflex and help support the digestive system. Aloe Vera juice can be taken in the morning and night. By adding a Digestive enzyme and a Probiotic to your diet daily will also help. As we get older our digestive system gets depleted and needs a little help. Also by rubbing with the pinky side of your right hand under your left breast side to side will stop this immediately. There is a point under your left breast that will be sore if your stomach is out of balance. Rubbing this point will help to bring the body back into balance.

## **Inflammation in the body**

Some signs of inflammation in the body are brain fog, memory impairment, ache and pains, mood issues.

Here is good drink for inflammation in the body.

8 oz of warm or hot water
1 tsp real maple syrup
½ of an organic lemon juice
½ to 1 tsp Organic Turmeric spice

Mix together and drink like a tea. You can drink this everyday to help with inflammation in the body.

Foods that help fight inflammation are tomatoes, strawberries, oranges, blueberries, cherries. Leafy greens like spinach, kale and collards. Nuts like almonds, walnuts. Fatty fish like salmon, mackerel, sardines, tuna and olive oil.

Stay away from fried foods, sodas, refined sugars, lard and processed meats.

Turmeric capsules are good to take also if you are having inflammation problems.

**To help clear inflammation in the Digestive system you could use:**

1 tsp of Turmeric spice and 1 cup of warm milk at bedtime

This will help with any inflammation in the colons and intestines.

Another way to stimulate and get the digestive muscles working again is to eat 1 stalk of celery and about ½ cup of blueberries between meals. This will help the muscles get back in shape.

## Clearing Parasites

*Take Black walnut, Clove and Wormwood Tincture before bed in 1 tablespoon of water three days before the full moon, on the full moon and 3 days after the full moon. It will tell you on the bottle how many drops to take.*

This works because Black Walnut and Wormwood kills the adults and the Cloves kills the egg of the parasite.

Everybody has parasites in their body. It's a good practice to do this before the full moon. You can get parasites tincture cleanses on Amazon or at your health food store. The combination tinctures work very well.

## Detoxifying

It is very important to keep your body clean from pollutant in the environment, food and water. Here are some of the remedies that I use to keep my body clean.

Archangel Michael said that we need to bless our food before we eat it and say over your food. 88-88-88-88 and hum the tone G. This will change the vibration of the food to be healthier for your body. When saying the eights, its eight - eight pause, eight - eight pause, eight - eight pause, eight -eight pause, then hum the tone G.

## Apple Cider Vinegar

Mix 2 tsp of Braggs Apple cider vinegar with 1/8 tsp Baking Soda in 8 ounces of water. Drink this first thing in the morning. This will help your body stay alkaline so your body can heal faster. You can also cut up a lemon and add it to the mixture.

## Epsom Salt and Clay Baths

Any kind of bath salts like Himalayan salts plane or with Essential oils are good.

Taking an Epsom salt or a clay bath every month is very helpful in detoxing your body. I use 1-2 cups of Epsom salts in a bath tub of water. Soak for 20 minutes.

When I am soaking, I imagine that I am in the purple water and all the toxins are coming out of my body thru my skin. You can buy Epsom salts at any store. They are very inexpensive.

I also use Pascalite Clay Powder from Wyoming. This is a wonderful product. I use ¼ of a cup in my bath tub. This is very good to remove heavy metals from the body. Soak for 20 minutes in the clay. When you are done and empty the water, you can see the metal flakes on the bottom of the tub.

If you are not able to soak in a bath tub, soak your feet. I would use about ¼ of the amount that you would use in the tub and soak for 20 minutes. When using a foot massage detoxer be careful and don't use it to much because it can deplete you of essential minerals. Emergen-C vitamin pack that you add water to contains vitamin and minerals to replenish the body. I drink this every day. It's simple, easy and tastes good.

# PectaSol-C

PectaSol-C is a supplement by Eco-Nugenics that has many benefits.

- Supports Cellular Health
- Supports a healthy Immune System
- Removes toxic Heavy Metals

This supplement is a natural product derived from the pith of citrus fruit peels, including lemons, limes, oranges, and grapefruits. I order this on-line. If you our experiencing a metal taste in your month you need this product.

# Himalayan salts

*Himalayan salts have many uses from cooking, clearing negative ions in the air using the lamps and using them in bath water. I place about 3 rocks with purified water in a pint glass jar with a plastic cover over the top. With a plastic spoon I drink 1 tsp of this in 8 oz glass of water every other day.*

*This contain trace minerals needed in the body, rich in iron, balances alkaline/acidity in the body, dissolve and eliminate sediment in the body.* This is so simple but has wonderful benefits for the body

# *Conclusion*

My prayer for all of you is that you find relief in whatever you are dealing with. Everything in this book has helped me and my clients in miraculous ways. If you are in a health crisis don't be afraid. Trust your inner guidance to get you through this. Your body is designed with everything that you need to heal and you have access to all the help that you need. Now go inside and ask God for what you need. People will show up to help you like Sr. Dorothy showed up for me.

The right people like Doctors, Healers, Natural Paths, Chiropractors, Spiritual guides, Books, Vitamins, etc will come to you. Be open to what God is bringing you to help you heal.

Don't be afraid to ask God why? He will tell you and you will be able to move forward from this.

Ask Him what you need to heal. It could be as simple as diet.

May God bless your journey and remember to be open to what God is bringing you.

With Love and Gratitude;
Joanne

The Amazing You Healing Meditation is available for purchase on the website for $9.99.

Purchase products through Facebook; Joanne Hammons Healing

Website; energykinesiology1.vpweb.com/Home

# References

The Ancient Cookfire by Carrie L'Esperance

Touch for Health by John Thie,M.Ed

Heal your Life with Home Remedies and Herbs by Hanna Kroeger

The Cure for all Cancers by Hulda Regehr Clark, Ph.D.,N.D.

Hands of Light by Barbara Ann Brennan

The Living Insight study Bible by Charles R. Swindol

You can Heal your Life by Louise L. Hays

The Secret Language of your Body by Inna Segal

The Spiritual Warfare Book by Dr. David Jeremiah

The Power of the Praying Wife and Parent by Stormie Omartian

The Catholic Warrier Prayer Download from the book An Exorcist Tells his Story by Father Gabriele Amorth

Awaken to the Healer Within by Rich Work with Ann Marie Groth

Healing Crystals and Gemstones by Dr. Flora Peschek-Bohmer and Gisela Schreiber

PDR for Essential oils compiled by Essential Science Publishing for Young Living

Releasing Emotional Patterns with Essential Oils by Carolyn L. Mein, D.C.

Healed of Cancer by Dodie Osteen

www.marytv.tv to pray the daily Rosary from Medjugorje

## *Products*

R.W.Knudsen organic juices no sugars added

PectaSol-C by Eco-Nugenics

Pascalite Clay Powder manufactured in Wyoming

Braggs organic raw-unfiltered apple cider vinegar "with the Mother"

Emergen-C dietary supplement distributed by Alacer Corp.

Essential Oils by Young Living

Printed in the United States
By Bookmasters